Harold W. Preiskel
Overdentures Made Easy:
A Guide to Implant and Root Supported Prostheses

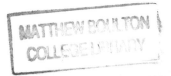

Overdentures Made Easy

A Guide to Implant and Root Supported Prostheses

Harold W. Preiskel

MDS (London), MSc (Ohio), FDS RCS (England)
Consultant, Dept of Prosthetic Dentistry
The United Medical and Dental Schools
of Guy's and St Thomas's Hospitals
Guy's Tower, London SE1 9RT

Quintessence Publishing Co Ltd
London, Berlin, Chicago, São Paulo, Tokyo, Moscow,
Prague and Warsaw

First published 1996 by
Quintessence Publishing Company Ltd
London, UK

© 1996 Quintessence Publishing Co Ltd

British Library Cataloguing in Publication Data
Preiskel, Harold W.
  Overdentures made easy: a guide to implant and root
  supported prostheses
  1. Overlay dentures   2. Implant dentures
  I. Title
  617.6'92

  ISBN 1-85097-039-4

Printed and bound by Toppan Printing Co Pte Ltd, Singapore
Litho production by JUP-Industrie- und Presseklischee, Berlin

Typesetting by Alacrity, Banwell Castle, Weston-super-Mare, UK

Introduction

Nearly a century has passed since the mathematician Sylvanus P. Thompson simplified calculus with a masterpiece that still represents the epitome of logical thought and clear writing. He pointed out that most authors feel obliged to impress their readers with their tremendous cleverness by solving problems in the most complex manner possible. They seldom show how easy it is to answer a straightforward question; yet if one masters the simple, the rest will follow. His remarks could hardly be more pertinent to prosthodontics today. Following his example, this text has been kept to a minimum and the reader is referred to other works for elaboration of subjects peripheral to the main theme.

The powerful weapon of osseointegration has introduced an entire new range of overdenture possibilities. This freedom of choice brings with it added responsibilities for the clinician, who must understand the similarities and important differences between root and implant supported restorations. While the importance of correct implant location and angulation has been stressed, surgical considerations of implant placement have not been included, as they are well covered in other books. For a similar reason, periodontal surgery is omitted. Since my own clinical experience is limited to one implant system, I am particularly grateful to Drs. Arvidson, Mericske-Stern and Geering, who have contributed their practical experiences with other well tried methods. The astute reader who detects a few small sections of repetition has not discovered a plot to enlarge the text; it is to avoid the annoying task of searching other chapters for cross references.

Some overdentures are quite easy to make, some can be extremely difficult. I hope that this book will help the reader anticipate problems, overcome obstacles, and master the basic technique of overdenture construction - the rest will follow!

Harold W. Preiskel
25 Upper Wimpole Street
London W1M 7TA

Foreword

George Zarb, B.CH.D. (Malta), D.D.S., M.S. (Michigan), M.S. (Ohio), F.R.C.D. (C), Dr. Odont. (H.C.), LL.D. (DAL), Professor and Head of Prosthodontics, Faculty of Dentistry, University of Toronto.

Overdenture treatment is a notion which precludes the inevitability of "floating plastic" in edentulous mouths. It has always offered a sensible and prudent appeal for dental practitioners, and numerous patients have benefited from its prescription. The applied ingenuity of the technique has mitigated much of the time-dependent risk inherent in the complete denture service – retention and stability are enhanced, residual ridge resorption retarded, and patient-mediated responses much improved. However, over-dentured abutments are vulnerable to infective processes, particularly in the context of the consequences of biological ageing. Consequently, the notion has not been prescribed to its fullest extent. The introduction of the so-called osseointegration technique by Schroeder, Branemark and other researchers has now tipped the therapeutic scale even further in the direction of the overdenture approach, because of an apparent less vulnerable response of osseo-integrated titanium tooth root ana-logues to a hostile oral milieu.

Several prosthodontists around the world refused to lose sight of the forest for the trees, and chose to develop the notion of implant suppor-ted overdentures rather than the de rigeur fixed option. As a result a new standard of prosthodontic service for the edentulous patient has emerged. I suspect it is only a matter of time before dental educators and practi-tioners will recognize the enormous merits of this newer and even more versatile notion.

Harold Preiskel has been at the forefront of promulgating the merits of the overdenture technique. His teachings and writings have been exemplary, and to his credit he was amongst the first to recognize the impact that osseointegration would have upon traditional removable prosthodontics. This book is the result, and we the readers will benefit enormously from the author's expan-ding repertoire. It is a lucid and informative text, sensibly argued, and a superb reconciliation of the basics of the overdenture notion with the advent of the osseointegration method. I feel very privileged to play a small part in this milestone publica-tion.

George Zarb

Acknowledgements

While it is impossible to list all who have helped with the development of this book, I would like to thank Drs. David Brown, B. Gillings, F.J. Kratochvil, Robert P. Renner, Pepe Tsolka, Julian Woelfel, George Zarb, and the late Dr. J.O. Forrest. The manufacturers of implants and attachment components have all been generous with their help. Miro Lavrin, Roy Yeatman, and Walter Thomas, are among those who have provided skilled technical work. Mrs. Gillian Lee drew the diagrams and the team in my practice have helped collect the photographs. The manuscript was produced, organised and arranged by Mrs. Elsie Crook. I am also grateful to Messrs. H.W. Haase, John Brooks and Joyce Ronald, together with the entire Quintessence staff, for their patient co-operation.

Contents

9

1   The development of the overdenture

An overdenture may be defined as a removable prosthesis that covers the entire occlusal surface of a root or implant. Such prostheses have found ever increasing applications in prosthodontics, which may be a reflection on population trends and the demand for better treatment. Surveys in most of the civilised world have shown that the percentage of those over 65 years of age is increasing, and statistics indicate that this trend will continue to the year 2000 and beyond as the post-war boom of babies grow older and move through society. Nowadays increasing age and the loss of teeth do not necessarily go hand-in-hand, but in the past, alveolar ridge resorption and a decrease in neuromuscular skills in manipulating complete dentures combined to detract from the quality of life of many patients.

Edentulousness, so long considered to be a normal part of ageing, can now be thought of as a disease entity.

Overdenture history

The idea of leaving roots of natural teeth to support an overdenture is far from new; even in 1856, Ledger had described a prosthesis resembling an overdenture. True, his restorations were referred to as plates covering fangs, and this became the title of a paper published by Atkinson some 5 years later. Indeed, following a conference in Connecticut in 1861 there appeared to be an increasing awareness of the value such roots might play in supporting a covering denture, while by 1888 Evans had described a method of using roots actually to retain restorations. In 1896 Essig had prescribed a telescopic-like coping. Peeso was also making what appeared to be removable telescopic prostheses at around the same time.

It was, of course, necessary to devitalise most of the roots employed and a great blow was delivered by William Hunter with his so-called focal sepsis theory (1909). A year later William Hunter delivered an address in Montreal describing present day restorative technique as "... a veritable mausoleum of gold over a mass of sepsis to which there is no parallel in the whole realm of medicine and surgery." Hunter's so-called focal sepsis theory had, therefore, spread to both sides of the Atlantic and his views were widely reported. As a result, wholesale removal of teeth was undertaken to treat diseases which, at the time, were of uncertain aetiology. Many years later, Rothman (1976) stated that Hunter's comments gave dentistry a black eye!

Continental Europe did not share the enthusiasm of Hunter and his disciples, so overdentures and similar constructions continued to be made. The reasons for retaining the roots were not always specified but it is likely that denture retention and stability must have been uppermost in clinicians' minds. Gilmore was obviously looking for both denture retention and stability, whereas Peeso (referenced in 1916) suggested that he was interested primarily in denture support. Most of the retention systems that were developed between the wars, and after the Second World War, provided support, stability and retention.

Advantages of preserving teeth or roots

Before considering implant overdentures some of the advantages of preserving roots should be considered as the effects are surprisingly similar. These can be considered under the following headings:

1. Psychological benefits to the patient.
2. Effects upon the edentulous ridge.
3. Tactile discrimination.
4. Improved stability and retention of the denture.

Psychological factors

The loss of remaining teeth can be a disturbing and emotional experience for many. Indeed, the stigmata and taboos of becoming edentulous have, in the past, overshadowed the practise of some forms of European dentistry to the extent of preserving rotten roots with purulent exudates around them. It may well be that loss of teeth is associated with ageing and this could be a depressive factor in some. Certainly the effects of body image, together with the emotions associated with the oral area, should not be underestimated. Reports on this aspect of therapy are generally anecdotal.

Effects upon the edentulous ridge

Bone is constantly remodelled and following loss of teeth, resorption of the alveolar ridge occurs. In 1967 and 1969 Tallgren showed that over a 7-year period the reduction of anterior ridge height of the mandible was four times greater than that of the maxillary edentulous ridge. However, Tallgren's 7-year studies of alveolar bone loss around mandibular natural teeth in patients with partial dentures showed the vertical loss to be only 0.8 mm, compared with a 6.6 mm loss in those wearing complete dentures. This difference in resorption rate will doubtless become more pronounced with advancing years. In 1978 Tallgren and others demonstrated the wide, and almost unpredictable, range of resorption patterns that may be found in patients 3 and 6 months after the insertion of immediate replacement dentures. Atwood and Coy (1972) corroborated Tallgren's findings of the 4:1 ratio of bone loss between mandibular and maxillary edentulous ridges. Crum and Rooney (1978), reporting a 4-year study, claimed that the retention of mandibular canines for overdentures helped preserve the remaining edentulous ridge. Their figures showed an average of 0.6 mm of ridge reduction in the anterior part of the mandible for patients with overdentures, whereas patients with complete dentures lost an average of 5 mm. Lord and Teel (1974) stressed that teeth too weak for normal partial denture abutments may be suitable for overdentures. Cutting down the teeth to just above mucosal level has a dramatic effect on crown root ratio – incidentally, it also facilitates plaque control. This type of approach is particularly useful when an otherwise edentulous ridge is opposed by natural teeth or a fixed prosthesis.

Tactile discrimination

Effective mastication which requires tactile discrimination relies upon feedback. The extraction of teeth should result in loss of mechanoreceptors from associated periodontal ligaments. Indeed, over the last 30 years a wide range of reports have all confirmed far greater discriminatory ability in dentate subjects compared with edentulous. Only the amounts vary from about 6 times the ability (Fenton, 1978) to 100 times (Kawamura and Watanabe, 1960). However, the feedback mechanism would appear to extend beyond the periodontal ligament, as anaesthetising the teeth appears to have little effect on discriminatory ability. This may be why patients with implant supported restorations appear to demonstrate such effective masticatory efficiency. After all, no periodontal ligaments exist around metal or ceramic root analogues.

Mericske-Stern has shown that the ability to perceive thin test foils placed between the artificial teeth of root supported mandibular overdentures was greater than those supported by implants. While receptors in the mucosa, proprioception in the muscles and TMJ may all influence discrimination, the periodontal receptors appear to play a significant role. However, there is no evidence to suggest that the improved tactile sensibility of roots positively contributes to individual chewing capacity, chewing comfort or maximal biting forces.

13

*Improved stability and retention
of dentures*

The vertical walls of the remaining root will provide some additional stabilisation for the overlying prosthesis. The greater the vertical space occupied by the root preparation, the greater the stabilisation provided. Implants produce stabilisation in a very similar manner, and the effect of this stabilisation along with a well made prosthesis can be quite surprising.

Additional retention is produced by parallel vertical walls of copings or by attachments. These retaining components will only produce long lasting effects if the prosthesis is fundamentally stable.

Drawbacks of overdentures

There are surprisingly few drawbacks, provided overdentures are properly designed and constructed. Nevertheless, overdentures cover all the gingival margins so that plaque control and denture hygiene of a high standard are essential.

Unfortunately, patients who are candidates for overdentures have not normally excelled in these respects so that careful explanation of the problem is vital. Overdentures cost more than complete dentures due to the endodontic and periodontal therapy required together with the root surface preparations involved. The abutment roots must possess a sufficiently good prognosis to justify this expenditure. Overdentures are bulkier than many other restorations. They would not normally be considered as alternatives to fixed prostheses except on grounds of cost. However, their bulk is greater than that of a removable partial denture and when the overdenture is removed at night the patient appears virtually edentulous. There is one other complication. Patients wearing overdentures may apply more load to their prostheses than complete denture wearers, yet the inherent strength may be less due to the space occupied by the root preparations (Fig. 1.1). Overdentures need to be planned with care.

The prognosis of the restoration is likely to be influenced by numerous factors, including the selection of the patient, treatment planning, preparation of the mouth, execution of the prosthodontic therapy and also by the maintenance therapy necessary to ensure a satisfactory result. Once this is appreciated, the way is clear to providing a useful and worthwhile overdenture service from which the patient will derive considerable benefit.

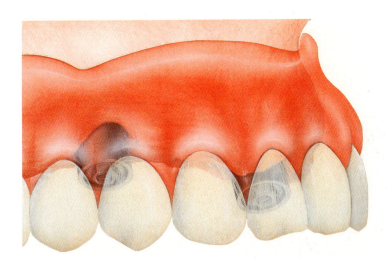

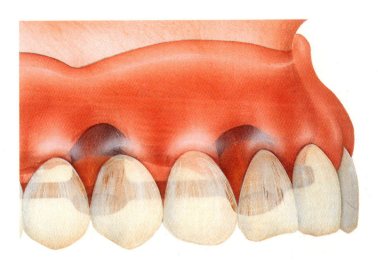

Fig. 1.1. Overdentures are inherently weaker than complete dentures made in a similar manner, due to the space occupied by abutments and the superstructure. However, the loads applied to an overdenture are likely to be greater.

Types of overdentures

Overdentures can be considered prostheses that cover teeth, roots, or implants, together with the edentulous ridges. This book is concerned with the application of complete overdentures, although other types will be described; four types of overdentures are mentioned:

1. Transitional overdentures.
2. Training overdentures.
3. Immediate replacement overdentures.
4. Definitive prostheses.

Transitional overdentures

This particularly useful group has application when the patient is already wearing a partial denture. The transitional overdenture consists of a modification of this partial denture to replace further lost teeth or to cover the roots of overdenture abutments once the teeth have been cut down (Fig. 1.2).

Training dentures

Strictly speaking, these are not overdentures, but they do have many applications in overdenture techniques. Such dentures are commonly employed to replace hopeless posterior teeth once they have been extracted. They serve as a replacement to allow the patient to accommodate to the replaced posterior dentition and to palatal coverage in the case of an upper restoration. This accommodation by the patient includes swallowing, chewing and speech patterns.

Immediate replacement overdentures

Immediate replacement overdentures are constructed before the last remaining teeth are extracted and the overdenture abutments prepared. A training denture is often converted to an immediate replacement overdenture that may, with judicious relining, be employed for several months, or years. Even when they are replaced, such prostheses may serve as spare dentures later on (Fig. 1.3).

Definitive prostheses

These restorations are usually constructed at least 6 months following extraction of the last teeth and the preparation of the overdenture abutments (Fig. 1.4). By the time such dentures are made, the edentulous ridges should be matured and the gingival margins firmly established. Dentures of this type may involve metal bases and some may be retained by attachments. They should be planned to provide service for several years.

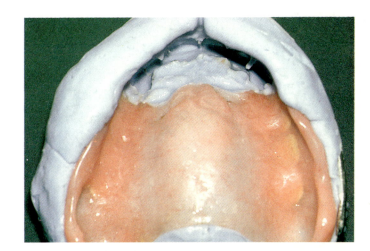

Fig. 1.2. A modified partial denture can be used as a transitional overdenture.

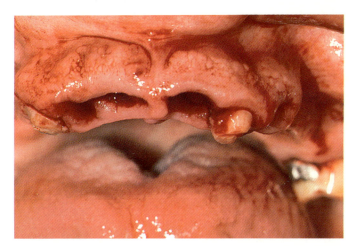

Fig. 1.3. Immediate replacement overdentures may be employed not only for the post-extraction period, but may serve as a spare denture later on.

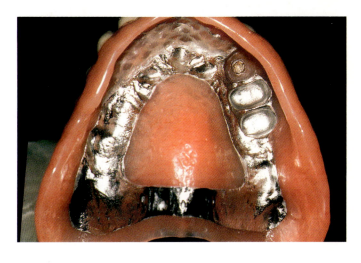

Fig. 1.4. Definitive overdentures are normally constructed some 6 months following extraction of the last teeth. Where implant supported prostheses are involved, they may be constructed from the outset.

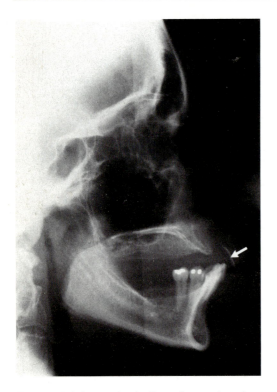

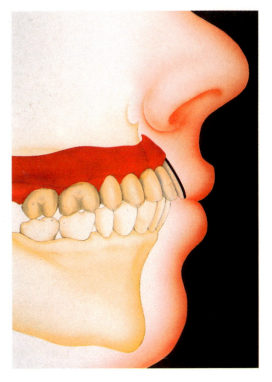

Fig. 1.5.(a) Lateral skull radiograph of a patient wearing a complete denture. A gutta percha point has been placed on the facial surface of the central incisor. Note the relationship of the facial skeleton to the artificial tooth position.

Fig. 1.5.(b) Diagrammatic representation of the radiograph.

Overdentures on implants

Overdentures supported by implants are a comparatively new arrival on the prosthodontic scene. It was only the development of well researched implant systems, providing a predictable success rate that made such restorations feasible. Initial results now suggest that when an implant is osseointegrated, marginal bone loss is reduced to levels that one would expect to find around healthy teeth. Marginal bone loss may be slightly greater around implant supported overdentures compared with implants supporting fixed prostheses, but apart from the first year, the bone loss levels compared with an edentulous jaw are dramatically improved. This, in itself, is a major factor in considering implant placement today.

Although most of the descriptions in the text will refer to the Branemark system, the principles apply to most

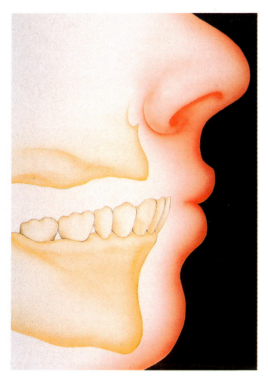

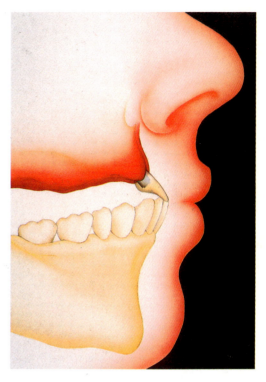

Fig. 1.6. Diagrammatic representation to show the relationship of the lips to the facial skeleton.

Fig. 1.7. Facially inclined implants cannot compensate for the loss of bone. This loss can only be corrected by a graft.

of the other established devices. Compared with an implant supported fixed prosthesis, an overdenture requires somewhat less support, offers far more flexibility in tooth positioning, seldom causes speech difficulties, and is more economical. On the other hand, it requires more maintenance, and is likely to be more difficult to construct, although these complications are seldom appreciated. Overdentures must be designed to withstand loads applied over long periods of time under a wide range of different loading conditions. The potential excessive bending moments applied to the implants are considerable, and it is hardly surprising that so many workers have reported complications with maintenance therapy. It has become apparent that implants are particularly susceptible to overload, and especially to forces that are non-axial.

Zarb has pointed out that using

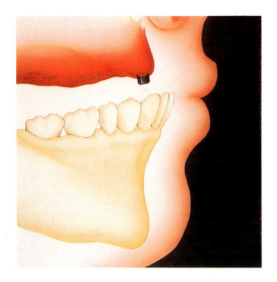

Fig. 1.8. A vertically aligned implant.

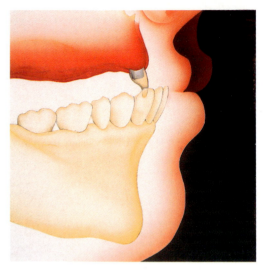

Fig. 1.9. A fixed prosthesis made on a vertically aligned implant will neither support the lips nor provide a correct relationship with the opposing jaw.

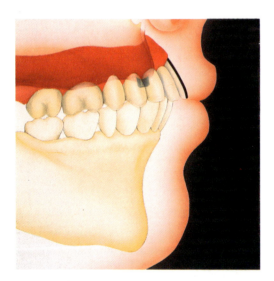

Fig. 1.10. An overdenture is an effective, neat and relatively economical method of restoring lip support without recourse to invasive or complex surgical techniques.

periodontal indices as a surrogate in assessing diseases around the implant is quite pointless, as there is no correlation. The elicited response from the same bacteria can be different from the periodontal ligament and from the tissues around the implant. Implants may be less susceptible to plaque-related diseases than roots. Constructing an overdenture supported by both roots and implants is normally ill-advised, as the operator has to face the drawbacks of both.

2 Treatment planning

Overdenture pitfalls

By the very nature of its construction, an overdenture covers the soft tissues surrounding the root or implant. The potential for plaque retention on the denture base is considerable, and an effective plaque control regime will be required to ensure a reasonable prognosis for the prosthesis and of its supporting structures. Since many overdenture candidates may not have enjoyed a distinguished record in this respect, plaque control instruction plays an important role in the initial therapy. Overdentures are space sensitive. It is seldom appreciated how important this vital aspect is to their construction. Both the intermaxillary space between the occlusal plane and the mucosa need to be considered. It is the space between the occlusal plane and the mucosa that determines the maximum dimensions of any restoration that is placed upon an abutment (Fig. 2.1). In the case of a maxillary implant where placement palatal to the crest of the ridge may be required, the entire contour of the anterior palate can be affected, to say nothing of the impingement of the opposing lower incisors. A similar effect can be produced by overzealous attachment placement on an anterior palatal root, which may well result in a subsequent denture fracture. Mandibular overdentures are no more straightforward, as there is minimal space to accommodate overbuilt abutments. Failure to assess space available is a common mistake and one of the most difficult to correct at a later stage (Fig. 2.2). This is why articulated diagnostic casts are so valuable.

A factor that we now have to consider is the site occupied by a potential abutment root. In days gone by, the alternatives were to consider an edentulous span or to make the best use of the root. Nowadays, we have the option of osseointegrated implants. In many intances where the prognosis of root abutments is dubious, we can now seriously consider replacing them with implants which should offer a far better prognosis – albeit at additional cost (Fig. 2.3). The sites are therefore

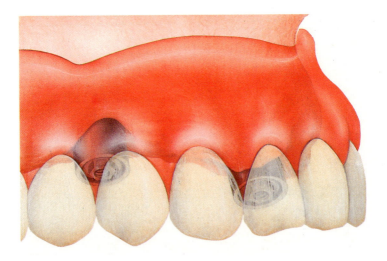

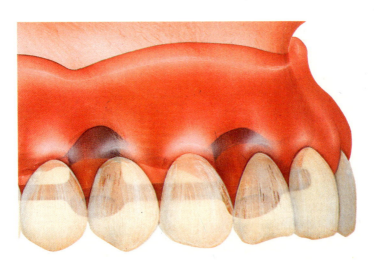

Fig. 2.1. The space between the occlusal plane and the mucosa determines the maximum dimensions of any restoration placed upon an abutment. One of the most valuable assets of treatment planning is a clear picture of the end result before treatment is actually begun.

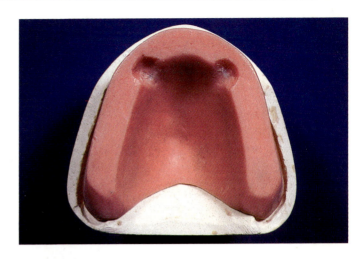

Fig. 2.2. When making jaw relationships for diagnostic casts, accommodate supra-erupted opposing teeth to allow for the correct establishment of the occlusal plane.

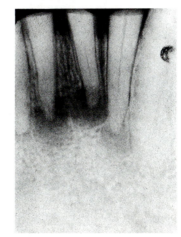

Fig. 2.3. A root with a dubious prognosis can now be replaced with an implant. The site may, therefore, be more valuable than the root occupying it.

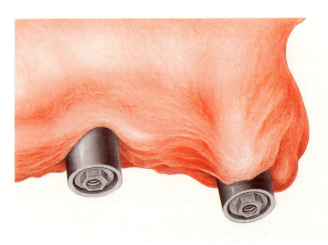

Fig. 2.4. Placing the implants before the tooth position has been established can be a hazardous procedure.

more valuable than the roots occupying them, a novel problem requiring thought and planning. Mixing roots and implants as overdenture abutments in the same jaw is not normally recommended.

Ōne of the most valuable assets in treatment planning is a clear picture of the end result before the treatment is actually begun. This image may be fairly straightforward where the patient presents with two or three teeth or roots. It is far more difficult to visualise when faced with an arcade of teeth, many with a hopeless prognosis. As for osseointegration procedures for an edentulous patient, it may well be temting to consider implant placement first and concern oneself with tooth position later on, but this is not the way towards an optimal result (Fig. 2.4). Step-by-step procedures are required but a clear image of the final result must be the guiding light throughout. Naturally, experience helps, but those with greatest expertise in the field are usually noted for the care that is taken with the preliminary stages of therapy. The importance of mounted diagnostic casts is apparent, together with the need to obtain all the information possible. While patients' wishes are paramount, such factors as support, available intermaxillary space and retention are key factors in the early planning stages (Fig. 2.5). When implants are to be considerd, a surgical stent made from an existing denture can provide a great deal of valuable information.

Overdentures on roots and implants present differing problems when the appearance is to be planned. Where roots are preserved, particularly canines, it is necessary to place the labial flange around the bony eminence that surrounds the root over an area that has not suffered significant resorption (Fig. 2.6). However carefully this is planned and executed, minor distortion of the sulcus must ensue and the extra prominence of the lip results in the lip line being raised and the patient showing more tooth. For maxillary overdentures, this will need to be accommodated by very slightly raising the incisal edges of upper teeth.

Implants are normally placed into a maxilla which has already resorbed significantly since the teeth were extracted, and the implant sites will be up to 1 cm palatal to the position that were occupied by the teeth (Fig. 2.7). The problem of distorting the labial flange does not apply in these instances but, conversely, there is the complication of producing a hump in the palate. The problems of appearance are less acute in most mandibular overdentures, although misplacement of implants facially will, of course, produce corresponding difficulties with the construction of the overdenture (Fig. 2.8).

A great deal of information can be obtained from the examination of an existing complete denture (Fig. 2.9). Using this prosthesis as a guide makes it easier to visualise the space available, taking into account the

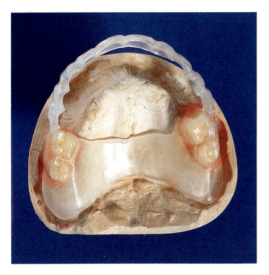

Fig. 2.5. Surgical stent made from an existing denture. Exaggerated facial position of the artificial teeth. Nevertheless, it can be seen that implants placed anterior to the canine region would produce unacceptable results unless the entire facial profile were changed.

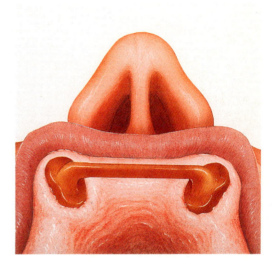

Fig. 2.6. Where roots are preserved, particularly upper canines, the bony eminence surrounding the roots is a complication. The labial flange will slightly distort the lip, while the absence of a flange will reduce both the stiffness and retention of the denture.

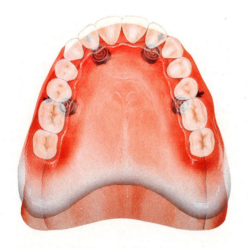

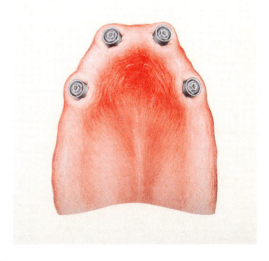

Fig. 2.7. Implants placed into a resorbed maxilla may be up to 1 cm palatal to the position originally occupied by the teeth. Unless care is taken with the superstructure, a hump can be produced distorting the shape of the anterior palate.

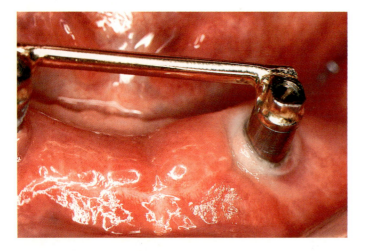

Fig. 2.8. The effect of placing a mandibular implant too far facially so that it is surrounded by mobile tissues. The problem is accentuated by poor plaque control.

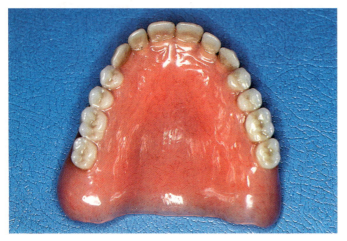

Fig. 2.9. Examination of the existing denture makes it easier to visualise the space available when implants are to be considered.

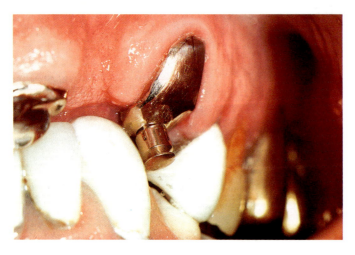

Fig. 2.10. Failure to assess vertical space available could lead to costly corrections. A preliminary assessment of vertical space and the occlusal plane will prevent this type of mishap.

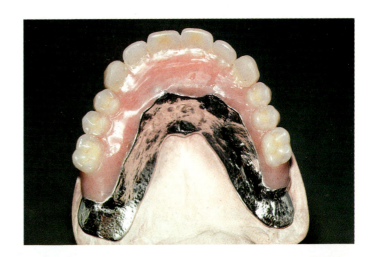

Fig. 2.11. An overdenture on implants can be made without a palate if four implants have been employed. However, such dentures exhibit high midline strain values so that a metal casting is essential.

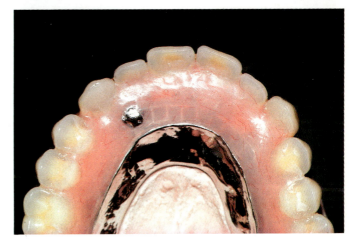

Fig. 2.12. An occlusal stop may be built into the metal casting where space is limited.

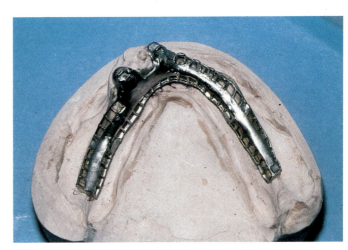

Fig. 2.13. The design of the tagging and the space for any attachments required cannot be left to chance.

need for a transmucosal abutment, precious metal coping and super-structure. For example, a complete maxillary denture with a thin palate bearing the imprint of lower incisors on the denture base covering the implant site does not bode well (Fig. 2.10).

Overdentures need to be designed to withstand a widely varying range of loading conditions applied over long periods of time. Dentures construct-ed entirely of acrylic resin are simpler and cheaper to produce, but exhibit far greater degrees of functional deformation when the buttressing effect of a flange is lost. If a horseshoe-shaped maxillary denture is considered for implants, a metal casting is essential to overcome the high midline strain values (Fig. 2.11). This factor is accentuated if the stiffness of the prosthesis is further compromised by large projections above the mucosa to accommodate abutment restorations or superstruc-tures placed upon implants. At least four implants are normally required before such an approach is con-templated.

Designing the metal framework can-not be left to chance. When attach-ments are to be incorporated a space must be provided to allow an ade-quate thickness of acrylic resin to surround the retaining unit. Where vertical space is restricted, usually in the palate, the metal casting may need to become the occluding sur-face as covering any metal structure with a paper thin layer of acrylic resin

in occlusion is a prescription for fracture (Fig. 2.12). Where bar re-tainers are used, maintenance is far simpler if the retaining clips are covered by acrylic resin rather than metal.

Another factor to bear in mind is the design of the tagging for mechanical attachment of the acrylic resin to the denture base (Fig. 2.13). In areas where rebasing may be required, such as the anterior palate, a spaced latticework design should be em-ployed. Where close adaptation between the denture base and the underlying mucosa is necessary, then the retaining system should take the form of small beads applied on the occlusal aspects of the cast.

Although the decision to make a metal denture base is one to be made at the treatment planning stage, the final contours of the casting can only be decided after the trial insertion. It is a very important feature to ensure that the artificial teeth are in the correct position before metal cast-ings are made. Attempting the con-struction the other way round is a gamble which often misfires.

Preparing the patient

Most patients appreciate careful and sympathetic explanation of the pro-posed treatment. It is an excellent means of establishing rapport be-tween operator and patient. On the other hand, lack of planning can cause a great deal of frustration and embarrassment. Other problems arise as a result of poor communication, as it is essential to relate the patient's expectations with what is actually feasible. For example, the prognosis of most overdentures and their abutments is best if the overdentures are removed at night. Ten minutes frank discussion at the beginning of treatment is worth more than hours of explanations and excuses at the end.

Cutting a tooth down to gingival level is a simple procedure; building it up subsequently is a very different proposition. Imagine the consequences of cutting teeth down to gingival level and then finding insufficient space for the overdenture that had been promised, and it can be understood why mounted diagnostic casts are invaluable planning aids.

To some patients, the emotional impact of tooth loss can be devastating, particularly if the patient is under considerable stress in the domestic or work environment. Establishing rapport is essential. It is a great mistake to proceed with prosthodontic therapy unless one is sure that the patient will co-operate fully with the treatment. At this stage it might be helpful to explain in some detail the way in which the therapy will be undertaken, stressing the patient's responsibilities with plaque control, home care and any other additional treatment that may be required.

Maintenance of overdentures is essential and the patient must be made aware that the structure of the mouth will change with time and will necessitate readaptation of the denture bases. Furthermore, mechanical gadgets may wear, or even break. Some repair will be required. Maintenance therapy is not simply normal; it is essential.

Examination and diagnosis

The following are intended as short notes to cover points commonly overlooked. They are not intended as a comprehensive list.

Medical history

The dental practitioner must be concerned with the general wellbeing of his patient, although prosthodontic therapy can be carried out even upon moderately sick patients should the need arise.

Heart disease

Patients with heart disease are probably the most common group at risk. Those with valvular disturbances usually require antibiotic protection against bacterial endocarditis. Others may be on anticoagulant or antihypertensive therapy, and it is therefore essential practice to work in co-operation with the patient's physician.

Hepatitis

Apart from the potential hazards to the patient during therapy, the dentist must be aware of possible dangers to himself and to other patients. Hepatitis B, also known as serum hepatitis, is diagnosed by detection in the blood of Australia antigen, now more commonly called hepatitis B antigen. The antigen is present in the saliva of serum positive patients and the virus could be transmitted from the patient to the dental surgeon. It is also possible for a dental surgeon who is unaware that his blood group is positive to infect his patient. In order to reduce risk to himself, the dentist should be wary of patients with a history of jaundice, multiple blood transfusions and renal dialysis. Since a vaccine is now available, it seems a sensible measure for all health care personnel.

AIDS

Although less infective than hepatitis, the consequences of a mishap are far more serious. Barrier techniques that are normally employed today should be sufficient to prevent accidental infection.

Debilitating medical and psychiatric disorders

Planning treatment here is usually a question of common sense. In most situations one would gear therapy to minimise the number of visits required and simplify maintenance as much as possible.

Strokes or any other medical complications that compromise the patient's ability to manipulate a prosthesis or to maintain an adequate level of oral hygiene require extra care in planning.

Dental history

Much useful information can be gleaned at this point, so it is important to establish rapport with the patient. Among the points of information to be obtained are the following:

1. Why did the patient lose teeth?
2. What was the success or failure of earlier prostheses?
3. What did the patient expect from previous prostheses?
4. Is the patient presently wearing a denture?
5. Is there any history of craniomandibular disorders?
6. Are there any home care difficulties?

It is apparent that patients who are already wearing dentures and who demonstrate a good level of oral hygiene are far easier to treat than others.

Examination

A thorough examination should be made of the oral cavity, teeth, edentulous areas and tongue.

Visual examination

Apart from the history, many would argue that visual examination is the most important part of the investigation. Among the items to note are:

General appearance.

Facial asymmetry.

Lip support.

Swellings or change of colour of the soft tissues.

The size and colour of the tongue.

The state of the periodontal structures.

The state of the remaining dentition, including the number, distribution, angulation and relationships of the remaining abutments.

The vertical and buccolingual space available for denture construction.

The contours of the edentulous ridges and denture bearing areas.

Digital examination

This important check includes palpation of any swollen areas, together with all the edentulous and denture bearing areas. Probing depths should be measured and the mobility of the teeth charted. Individual teeth should be checked for caries, and the margins of existing restorations assessed, while the temporomandibular joints should be palpated during opening, closing and lateral movements. If there is an anomaly, a transitional prosthesis may be required until a normal range of jaw movements has resulted.

Radiographic examination

Extra-oral and panoramic techniques such as those obtained with a Panelipse or Orthopantomograph are useful screening methods for all patients. However, they are not a substitute for a set of full mouth paralleling technique intra-oral radiographs that will provide accurate information that will help with the selection of abutments.

Implant therapy will require more specialised techniques. For the mandible anterior to the mental foramen, the operator may be prepared to accept an orthopantomagram provided that the distortion of scale can be calculated – usually with a radio opaque marker of known dimensions (Fig. 2.14). Careful bimanual palpation will be required to check for concavities, particularly those on the lingual aspects of the jaw. Elsewhere, CT scans are normally recommended, although the Scanora technique gives excellent results at lower cost (Fig. 2.15). The value of a CT scan is enhanced by modern programmes such as Dentascan and Columbia, which provide the operator with unrivalled information. Although radiation dosage is relatively high, the beam is closely collimated.

The Scanora system is another valuable adjunct to treatment (Fig. 2.16). It should provide accurate cross-sections of select areas with less radiation and considerably less cost than comparable CT scans and has the further advantage that the presence of metallic restorations does not cause the dispersion pattern seen with some of the earlier CT programmes. For localisation in large edentulous areas, a stent with radio-opaque markers may be required

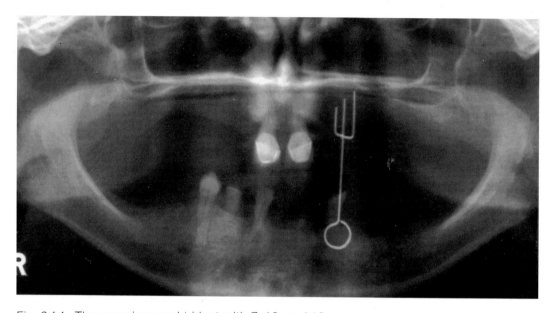

Fig. 2.14. The superimposed trident with 7, 10, and 13 mm projections serves as a guide to compensate for distortion.

Fig. 2.15. The value of a CT scan, enhanced by programmes such as Dentascan or Columbia, provides the operator with unrivalled information.

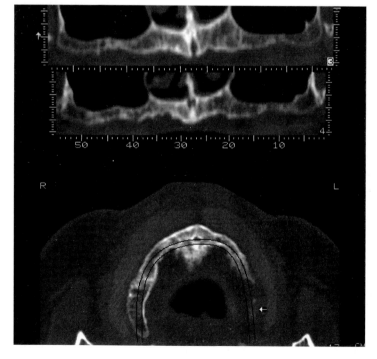

Fig. 2.15.(a)

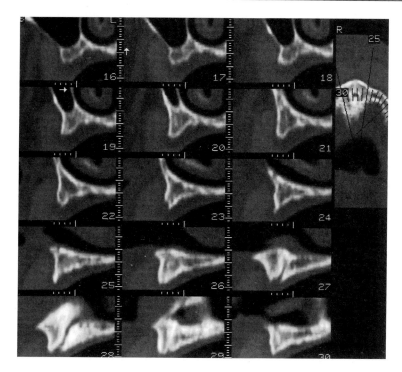

Fig. 2.15.(b)

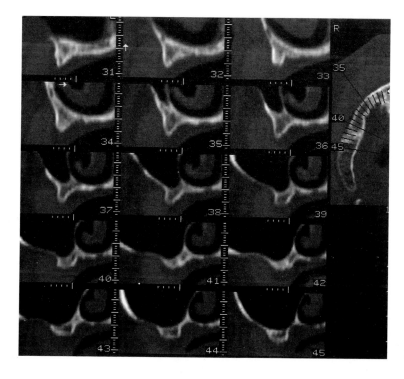

Fig. 2.15.(c)

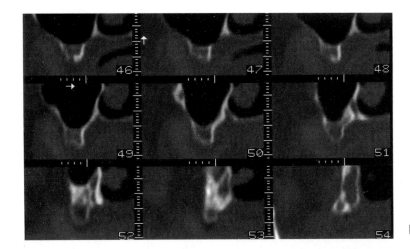

Fig. 2.15.(d)

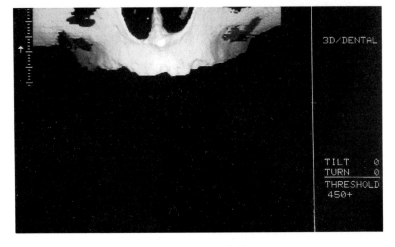

Fig. 2.15.(e)

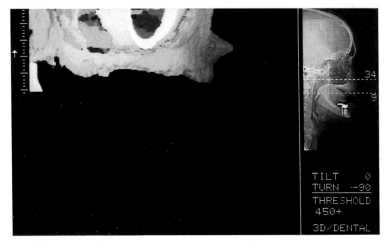

Fig. 2.15.(f)

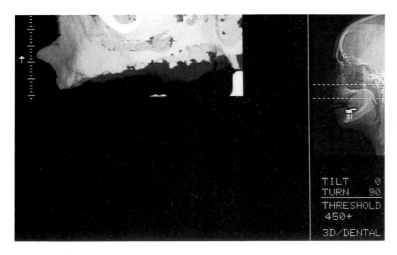

Fig. 2.15.(g)

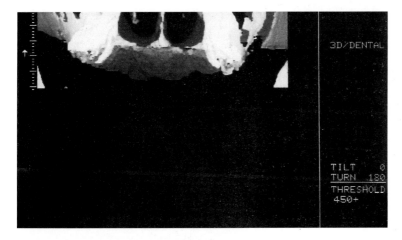

Fig. 2.15.(h)

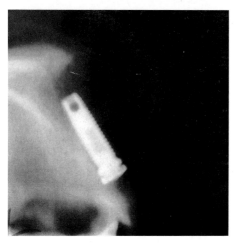

Fig. 2.16. Scanora view of anterior maxilla showing implant facially placed.

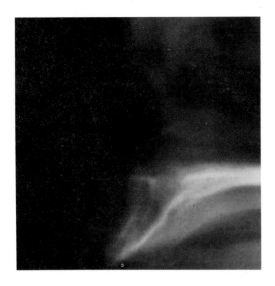

Fig. 2.17.(a) Scanora cross-section of maxilla. (b) Scanora view of premolar region. (c) Scanora view of posterior maxilla (different patient).

Fig. 2.17.(a)

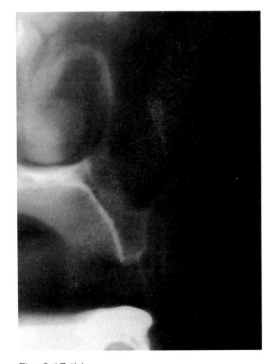

Fig. 2.17.(b)

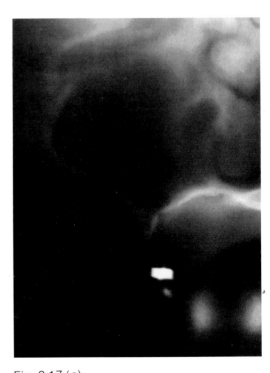

Fig. 2.17.(c)

The images produced are magnified and the use of the manufacturer's suitably calibrated ruler makes interpretation far more straightforward (Fig. 2.17).

The success or failure of most restorations can usually be judged by the state of the periodontium. For overdentures the periodontium is a critical region, but the whole mouth is, of course, involved.

While a provisional treatment plan will have been made at the outset some modification may have been necessary. A revised plan of action might be:

1. Emergency care.
2. Selection of abutments.
3. Disease control (caries and periodontal disease).
4. Extraction of hopeless teeth.
5. Endodontics.
6. Transitional or training partial dentures.
7. Periodontal surgery, and recontouring of denture bearing areas when necessary.
8. Waiting period for tissue maturation, possibly 8–12 weeks.
9. Construction of overdentures.
10. Maintenance therapy.

Pretreatment records

Among the most useful pretreatment records are mounted diagnostic casts. These casts, mounted on a suitable articulator, facilitate analysis of the occlusion, deflective contacts, tooth positions and angulations, jaw relationships and contours of the denture bearing areas and the space available for dentures. Furthermore, one can select a suitable path of insertion, determine undercuts relative to the pathway, and plan the arrangement of artificial teeth.

Photographs

Colour transparencies showing the arrangement of the remaining teeth and the state of the surrounding tissues can be particularly helpful. Some operators use profile photographs to help with assessment of the vertical relation of occlusion and of lip contour.

Additional measurement of vertical space

A simple measurement can be made with a pair of dividers, placing them on the gingival margin of the opposing teeth when they are in occlusion. This measurement is simply recorded on the patient's treatment card.

Consultation with other specialists

The periodontist, endodontist and oral surgeon are most likely to be the specialists whose expertise will be needed. The earlier they are consulted, the sooner a treatment plan may be established and implemented.

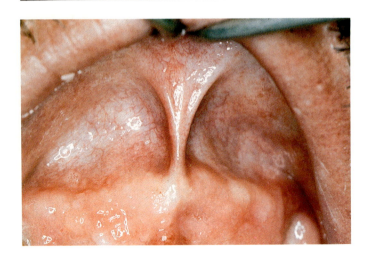

Fig. 2.18. A large labial frenum that will require reduction.

Diagnosis

The information obtained will form the basis for the diagnosis. Rampant caries is almost a disease of the past, although root decay in elderly patients continues to cause problems. Chronic periodontitis will be the most common cause for tooth loss today. In addition, there may be congenital problems, occlusal complications or even accidents that require overdenture therapy. It is, however, important to make a diagnosis – obvious as it may appear to be.

Overdentures may be considered if four or fewer retainable sound teeth are present in one arch. Complete dentures would be preferable for disinterested and unco-operative patients. Younger patients, particularly, benefit from overdenture construction.

The transitional phase of overdenture construction

In planning overdenture construction, one must not forget the difficult transitional phase facing the patient. Modern society makes it unacceptable to leave a patient without anterior teeth during any lengthy phase of denture construction.

Hopeless posterior teeth should be extracted as soon as possible and preferably at least 6 weeks before prosthodontic therapy. Reduction of a large overcontoured tuberosity or labial fraenum should be carried out at this stage (Fig. 2.18). It is the removal of hopeless anterior teeth that causes the problems, particularly as sound anterior teeth will require preparation involving cutting them down to just above gingival level.

Endodontic therapy to the sound abutments should have been com-

Fig. 2.19. If the patient is already wearing a partial denture this can be modified to act as a transitional prosthesis. A partial denture such as this can only be improved upon. Ideally, hopeless posterior teeth should be extracted and the sockets allowed to heal before overdenture construction is commenced.

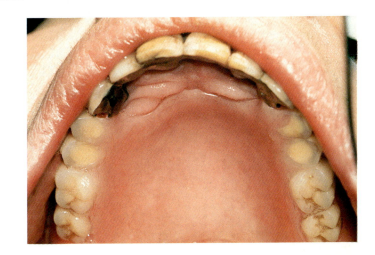

Fig. 2.19.(a)

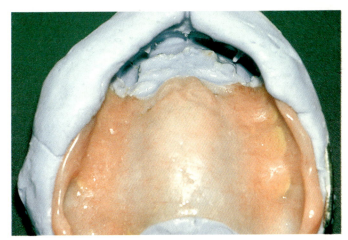

Fig. 2.19.(b)

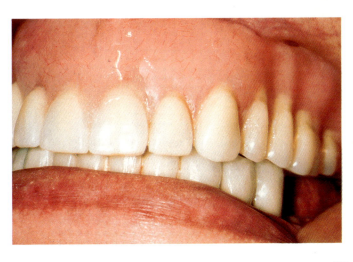

Fig. 2.19.(c)

pleted during the initial healing phase of the posterior teeth sockets. Planning of the next stages of therapy can be divided into situations where:

1. The patient is already wearing a partial denture.
2. The patient has no partial denture.

The treatment is considerably simplified when the patient already wears a partial denture. Adaptation to wearing a prosthesis will have occurred and this will be a great help in the transition to an overdenture. Posterior teeth may be added to this partial denture in the conventional manner. The prosthesis is placed in the mouth and an overall impression made in an alginate material and the impression cast. The posterior teeth and the corresponding flange can be added on an immediate replacement basis. A similar approach can be employed for anterior teeth, although the patient would doubtless wish to wait while the laboratory procedures were undertaken.

Adding flanges to partial dentures, or even a complete palate to an upper partial denture, is an effective and very rapid method of producing a transitional prosthesis while the patient waits (Fig. 2.19). A modified approach of this method is particularly useful for individual abutment preparations. The partial denture is removed in an overall alginate impression and then the abutment teeth prepared. The area around the abutment teeth is protected with petroleum jelly, and self-polymeris-

ing tooth coloured acrylic resin is then placed in the alginate impression corresponding with the tooth concerned. The impression is then replaced in the mouth. This provides an accurate and simple method of adding tooth crowns or even replacing teeth. Using a similar procedure, it is possible to incorporate a fixed prosthesis into the partial denture, thereby converting it to a transitional overdenture.

Patients with no partial denture pose far more difficult planning problems, not least the adaptation to wearing a prosthesis. The problem here is naturally that of obtaining a satisfactory impression for a complete overdenture while still leaving sufficient teeth in place with which to retain a transitional restoration. This transitional prosthesis may be fixed or removable, depending on the patient's preference and the number and support of abutment teeth. The hopeless posterior teeth not involved in a transitional restoration are removed, but others that are hopeless may be left in the mouth and prepared to aid the support and retention of the transitional fixed prosthesis. The restoration is constructed using acrylic resin or empimine materials. This transitional restoration will need to be removed for impression, jaw relation and trial insertion procedures. This method of approach is particularly valuable if employed to spare integrating implant sites from loading. The impression for the overdenture is made over the prepared, but hopeless, abutments and the cast trimmed to replace these teeth with the conventional immediate replacement technique. When the overdenture has been constructed, the condemned teeth are removed and the prosthesis inserted over the sound abutment preparations. Retention is obtained by border seal together with adhesion and cohesion.

Roots that can be salvaged are treated slightly differently. The impression for the initial overdenture is made over the abutment preparations and these preparations are subsequently cut down to root facings at a later stage. In this way, some vertical and buccolingual space is provided for an attachment assembly if this is to be employed later on. Otherwise, the space in the denture can be obliterated with self-polymerising resin. This immediate replacement overdenture can be considered a trial prosthesis and adjustments to the border fullness are made while adapting the patient to wearing such a restoration. Later on, the abutments can be prepared for the overdenture, impressions made, and gold restorations inserted and luted.

It must be stressed that the path of insertion of any restoration or attachment must be aligned with that of the denture and so an impression of the entire arch is necessary even if the abutments concerned occupy only a small section of it. A certain amount of trial and error is inevitable in adapting the overdenture to the new underlying restoration, and disclosing materials such as Fit-Checker (G.C. Chemical Mfg. Co., 76 Hasunuma-cho, Itabashi-ku, Tokyo) are particularly useful for this purpose. In many instances, it would be unnecessary to incorporate the female attachment in this initial overdenture, the procedure being deferred until the definitive restoration is constructed some 3 months later. When the definitive overdenture has been made, preferably metal-based, the initial overdenture will serve as a very useful spare prosthesis.

Patients undergoing implant therapy pose different problems, as no load should be applied over the area of surgery for at least a week. Where the patient is edentulous it means that the complete denture cannot be worn during this period and it is apparent that the patient must be made aware of this complication when implant therapy is first discussed. For some, it will mean that implant therapy is simply not possible due to domestic relationships and the earlier this is discovered the better. In fact, should healing be delayed, the period without the prosthesis may need to be extended. This rule can be broken if the edentulous area is spanned by a tooth supported transitional fixed prosthesis that can be reinserted immediately following the operation. If a tooth supported removable partial denture is available, the operator must be confident that the implanted area is spared all load if the prosthesis is to be worn during the first few days.

Once the initial healing has taken place, the original denture may be completely cut away from the implant sites using a disclosing material as a guide and the prosthesis readapted using a tissue conditioning material. The patient will need to be examined the next day to ensure there are no signs of ulceration, and the lining material will require to be changed at regular intervals throughout the integration period.

Nevertheless, following implant placement it is likely that no denture could be worn for about a week if it covers the implant site. This rule can be broken if there are strategic implant or root abutments that ensure that no load can possibly be applied to the area of surgery.

The stages of treatment

Once the initial investigations have been undertaken, it should be possible to divide the treatment into several well defined stages. While the operator may possess a clearly defined plan, it is all too easy to overlook the patient. That is why it is sensible to spend time explaining the stages of therapy, the time involved and the likely costs. Any changes in appearance should be clearly understood and if there is a period when the prosthesis cannot be worn this should be appreciated at the outset. The old adage still applies: "A few moments of explanation at the beginning is worth hours of excuses at the end". Examples of such plans are:

Patient A

1. Continuation of oral hygiene instruction, scaling and polishing.
2. Removal of hopeless posterior teeth and construction of a transitional or training denture.
3. Further oral and denture hygiene counselling.
4. Periodontal surgery, if necessary.
5. Endodontic therapy.
6. Insertion of immediate replacement overdenture.
7. Make a definitive overdenture. This may involve dental bases and/or attachments,

or

continue with an immediate replacement denture following rebasing

or

convert to a complete denture.

Patient B

1. Oral and denture hygiene instruction.
2. Construction of an immediate replacement complete denture.
3. Extraction of remaining teeth and insertion of denture.
4. Post-insertion adjustments.
5. After approximately 6 months, consider implant placement. Ex-

plain that a denture cannot be worn for at least a week following implant surgery.

6. Post-surgical modification of complete denture.
7. Construction of implant supported and retained overdenture. Examine possibility of converting the complete denture to a spare overdenture.
8. Post-insertion adjustments and maintenance.

Patient C

1. Oral hygiene instruction, scaling and polishing.
2. Selection of transitional abutments for a provisional resin fixed prosthesis. Extraction of infected and hopeless teeth.
3. Construction of provisional resin fixed prosthesis to span the edentulous areas to be restored.
4. Insertion of implants within interabutment spaces and replacement of provisional fixed prosthesis.
5. Construction of implant supported and retained overdenture and extraction of transitional abutments.
6. Post-insertion adjustments and maintenance.

The permutations and combinations of techniques available are enormous. In some instances hopeless roots can be employed as transitional overdenture abutments. Immediate insertion of implants following tooth extraction may be considered where the bulk of the implant is in fresh, healthy bone apical to the socket. Semi-permeable membranes and even grafts can be used but must be well shielded from load bearing. The only indispensable factor is a clear picture of the end result and a well focused plan of the route.

Summary

Planning the transitional phase is essential to the success of the entire treatment. Patients who have already worn a partial denture are normally easier candidates for overdenture construction and the transitional phase is far simpler. When an overdenture is the first denture a patient has ever worn, the double denture technique described has considerable advantages in allowing the operator to spend some time deciding upon and improving the appearance as well as accustoming the patient to an overdenture. Few patients experience significant problems with immediate insertion complications, provided adequate border seal can be obtained. A series of post-insertion appointments must be planned when plaque control and denture hygiene is stressed.

The metal-based definitive prosthesis can be made when healing of any extraction sockets has taken place.

3 Selection and preparation of abutment roots

This chapter is concerned with the selection of teeth or roots as overdenture abutments. In most situations the operator will have little choice, as there is seldom an abundance of abutment candidates. Indeed, should there be numerous potential abutments the overdenture may not be the ideal restoration. In making a decision the following points should be borne in mind.

Periodontal considerations

Reducing the tooth to gingival level drastically decreases the leverage ratio of forces inclined to the axial alignment of the root. However, the additional forces that might be applied through the overdenture require consideration.

Estimating the bone support around a root can be surprisingly difficult as bone levels are measured from radiographs. It is easy to overlook the conical shape of most roots. A cross-section of root near the apex will have a far smaller periphery than one closer to the amelocemental junction. When the height of the bone level has been reduced to half the normal amount, the loss of periodontal support is, therefore, far greater. Despite this complication, bone support will be discussed in terms of height as it is a method familiar to all clinicians.

Endodontic considerations

There is little point in making unnecessary complications. Sound teeth with satisfactory root fillings must obviously be strong candidates for abutment selection. Single rooted teeth are usually easier to root fill than multi-rooted teeth and should be given preference provided that bone support and other considerations are equal. Multi-rooted teeth can, of course, be considered for overdenture abutments and hemisection techniques can be valuable.

Endodontic problems in the overdenture population

Where there is an abundance of secondary dentine, endodontic therapy may not be considered worthwhile particularly if thimble shaped

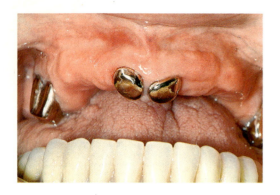

Fig. 3.1. Overdenture abutments opposing natural teeth or osseointegrated fixed prostheses will have a beneficial effect on the adjacent edentulous ridge.

copings are to be produced. Ettinger in 1990, reporting on a series of studies, showed that the most common cause of abutment failure (53.8%) was vital teeth developing periapical lesions as a result of pulp necrosis. Recurrent caries accounted for 23.1% of abutments lost and other failures included vertical root fractures. Although there was no detectable exposure in the vital teeth, it is apparent that these abutments were at risk, with nearly 15% developing complications. It was hypothesised that cutting the teeth down might open micro exposures into the pulp and on average it took about three years for lesions to be recognised (Fig. 1). There is some evidence to suggest that secondary dentine does not form an absolute seal and it may be necessary to provide additional sealing agents even over calcified roots if they are to be cut down. Yearly radiographs are obviously important.

Number of overdenture abutment teeth

Two abutments on opposing sides of the arch, say in the canine regions, will provide excellent results, while four widely separated abutments are even better. More abutments can be retained, although the advantages are not so clear cut and the complexity of the construction increased. Furthermore, if there are a large number of abutment teeth available, the operator should consider carefully whether the overdenture is really the restoration of choice. At the other end of the scale, overdentures can be made where there is only one abutment, although this adds to the difficulty of obtaining a satisfactory result.

The amount of space between abutments

Adjacent roots can complicate plaque control and denture construction. Where inter-radicular

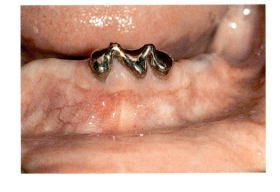

Fig. 3.2. Connecting copings offers mechanical advantages at the expense of complicating plaque control and denture construction. Sufficient interradicular space is essential.

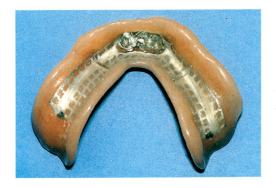

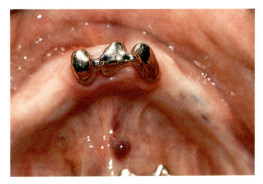

space is particularly restricted, removal of the weaker root may be worthwhile. If adjacent roots are to be preserved, the simplest approach is to restore each of the two surfaces with individual copings.

Connecting the root surfaces has several mechanical advantages. Inclined loads may be resolved into a more axial direction and there will be a marked resistance to loads with a lateral or rotational component (Thayer and Caputo, 1980). It is the need to provide adequate space for cleansing under the connection that is the problem. The connection will need to be swept up away from the gingivae and this in turn will complicate the design and construction of the overlying denture. This method will only work if there is sufficient space between the abutments to permit adequate plaque control of the proximal surfaces. It is an approach that may be employed when an attachment is positioned on one of the roots (Fig. 3.2).

Teeth present in the opposing arch

All other factors being equal it is normally wise practice to select overdenture abutments opposing remaining natural teeth.

A well known clinical finding is fibrous replacement of a maxillary ridge opposing six lower anterior teeth, if these teeth are the sole survivors in the mouth. If it is possible, preserve an upper root or two: the beneficial effects on the adjacent edentulous ridge will be considerable (Fig. 3.3).

Abutment preparation

The preparation of the abutment teeth is one of the keys to the construction of the overdenture. Assuming that the periodontal support is adequate, the operator has the choice of three approaches to the abutment preparation. The vertical space available is the main constraint, for it must be appreciated that whatever projects above mucosal level represents a corresponding depression or hole within the impression surface of the denture. The three basic approaches are (Fig. 3.4):

1. Preparation of the root surface just above mucosal level.

    (a) The bare root face.
    (b) The dome-shaped gold coping.

This approach occupies minimal space with the least influence on the path of insertion of the denture, least compromises the strength of the overlying denture but offers little additional stability and no extra retention.

2. The use of attachments.

    Intermediate in space requirements between the other two approaches, careful selection of the path of insertion, together with an assessment of the space available, is still required. Rebasing and repairs are normally more complex when attachments are employed, although the stability and retention they provide can be most valuable.

3. The thimble shaped coping.

    The thimble forms the inner section of a two-layered telescopic prosthesis. This approach occupies the greatest amount of vertical and buccolingual space and has a profound influence upon the denture design. Depending on the contours of the copings, a significant increase in both retention and support is offered.

Preparation of the root surface just above mucosal level

The bare root face.

There should be little question of leaving an irregularly shaped rough root surface as an abutment. The The occlusal section of the root

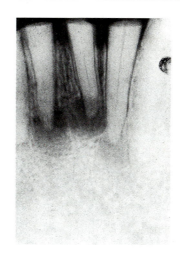

Fig. 3.3. Secondary dentine may not form an absolute seal and non-root filled abutments should be radiographed yearly to check for periapical changes.

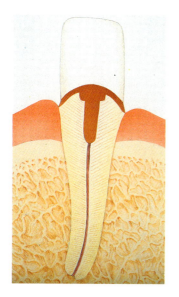 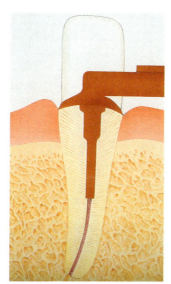 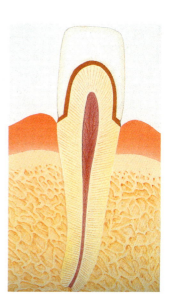

Fig. 3.4. Three types of abutment preparation: (a) Root face or gold coping just above mucosal level. (b) An attachment. (c) A thimble shaped coping.

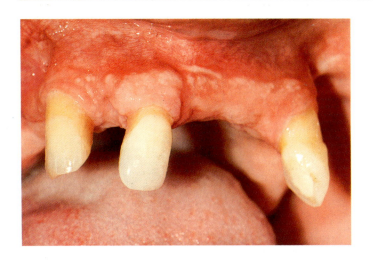

Fig. 3.5. Maxillary root filled teeth.

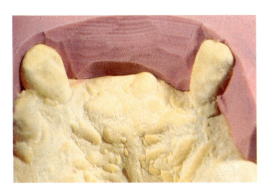

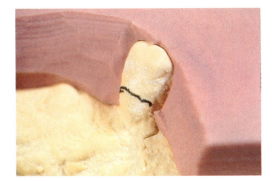

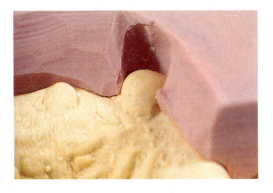

Fig. 3.6.(a) A silicone mask is a valuable aid in preparing the master cast. It preserves the outline of the facial and incisal edges of the abutments. (b) A pencil line is used as a guide to the initial reduction. (c) Following reduction, the space available for the abutment is clearly visible. Never over reduce the abutment.

canal can be obturated with a glass ionomer restoration or silver amalgam and if a curved and highly polished surface can be produced, the bare root abutment can be considered to have the following advantages:

1. It is the simplest, cheapest, and least space consuming solution.
2. It is the ideal solution during maturation of edentulous ridges following an immediate insertion technique, or while the gingival margins are becoming established following muco-gingival surgery.
3. This approach can also be used if time is required to evaluate questionable teeth or the co-operation of the patient.

Contra-indications

There are three principal contra-indications to leaving a bare root face:

1. It should not be used on a long term basis where natural teeth are in direct opposition. The incidence of longitudinal root fractures has been significantly raised in these circumstances (Bolender, Smith and Toolson, 1984).
2. Opposing bare root surfaces should not be left (Morrow, 1984). The dentine-to-dentine contact can produce a surprisingly high rate of wear.
3. Bare root surfaces should not be used on a long term basis unless a highly polished surface can be produced.

The bare root face approach is normally employed for immediate insertion prostheses, even if copings or attachments are to be employed at a later stage (Fig. 3.5). Whatever the final restoration, the initial reduction of the tooth follows a similar pattern – the golden rule being never to over-reduce. An immediate insertion restoration requires trimming of the master cast, a procedure that operators are strongly advised to do themselves until a definite understanding is reached with the laboratory (Fig. 3.6).

Over-enthusiastic reduction of the cast can lead to untold difficulties when an attempt is made to insert the prosthesis. Trim the cast so as to produce a convex root surface and then reduce the facial aspect further to allow room for the ridge lap of the artificial tooth. Err on the side of undertrimming the cast, as a small space between root surface and denture base can be obliterated with a carefully controlled application of self-polymerising resin. The gingivae and adjacent mucosa are protected with petroleum jelly and a small lingual vent cut so that excess material flows through it rather than under the denture base.

When crowned teeth are to be reduced, never make the mistake of attempting to cut under the gingival margin of the crown as this will lead to over-reduction (Fig. 3.7 a & b).

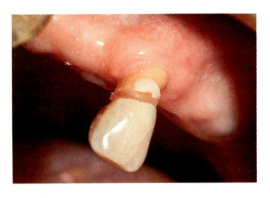 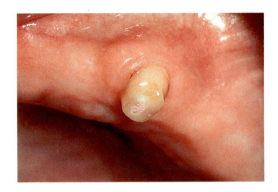

Fig. 3.7.(a) The initial cut through the root filled tooth. Always err on the side of leaving too much root substance. To avoid the risk of inhalation, do not cut entirely through the tooth but leave a very small portion intact. The crown is then broken off. An alternative method is to drill a hole through the crown and thread floss through it. (b) With the crown removed, the root preparation can be commenced.

Instead, cut through the crown or remove it and then reduce the underlying preparation like a tooth. For immediate insertion overdentures outline the root preparations before extraction of the hopeless teeth (Figs. 3.8– 3.11).

The precious metal coping

The operator has considerable scope with the design of the contours and may use the copings to connect adjacent roots. Single, unconnected, copings are normally produced, in view of the complications with plaque control that almost inevitably arise with even the best designed connections (Fig. 3.12). Connections also complicate the design of the over-denture and are reserved for situations where the mechanical advantages necessitate this approach.

Cutting root filled teeth down, and preparing dome-shaped copings that extend only 1 or 2 mm above the ridge crest, produces significant improvement in the crown/root ratio. Lateral loads are reduced and the space occupied is at a minimum. In this instance, the roots are being employed to give a measure of support against vertical loads, while their contribution to retention will be negligible (Fig. 3.13). The number and distribution of the roots, together with the adaptation of the denture to the root preparations, will determine their contribution to denture stability. This popular and effective method of preparing overdentures was developed by Lord and Teel (1969), with extremely satisfactory results. Since vertical space requirements are so small, the strength of the denture is virtually unaffected and breakages are relatively rare. In a survey of 250

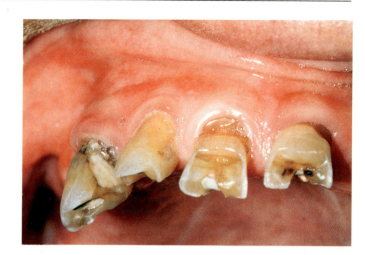

Fig. 3.8. Root filled teeth prior to immediate insertion of restorations.

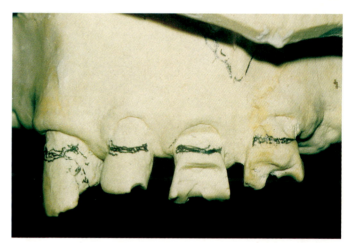

Fig. 3.9.(a) Plans for initial reduction of the master cast.

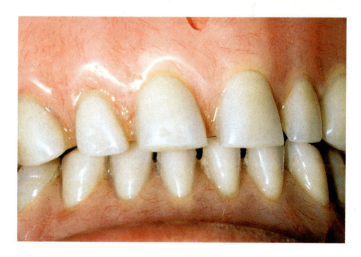

Fig. 3.9.(b) Restoration in place.

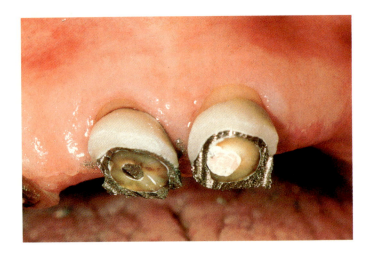

Fig. 3.10. When crowned teeth are to be reduced, either remove the crowns or cut through them. Never attempt to cut under the margins of the crowns, as this will over-reduce the abutments.

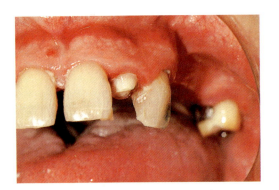
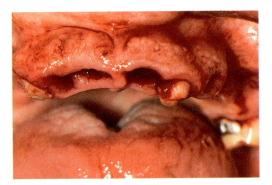
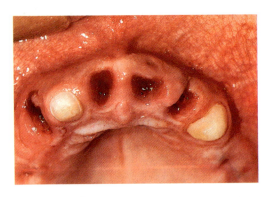
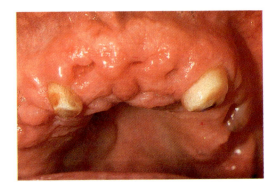

Fig. 3.11.(a)–(c) For immediate insertion of overdentures, outline the root preparations before extraction of the hopeless teeth. (d) Abutment following initial healing of extraction socket.

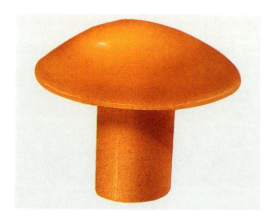

Fig. 3.12. Precious metal copings should be simple to clean.

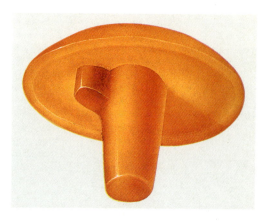

Fig. 3.13. Since no retention is being provided, relatively short dowels will suffice although anti-rotation components are essential.

overdentures, Reitz, Weiner and Levin (1977) found only one that had broken.

Because of the small lateral loads on the roots, this technique can be employed where lack of root support or vertical space precludes the use of telescopic thimble copings or attachments. Impression techniques and location procedures are simplified, as is plaque control. This type of approach may be used in conjunction with immediate replacement overdentures, since rebasing and relining techniques do not differ from those employed with complete dentures.

At one time, copings were recommended for immediate replacement dentures, but in view of the soft tissue changes that occur rapidly, these copings will need to be remade within a few months. Nowadays one normally leaves a bare root surface while the initial maturation of the edentulous ridge takes place and until the gingival margins have become finally established. This delay also provides the opportunity to re-evaluate the patient's plaque control. At this time, the abutment can be reprepared, the margins defined, and the coping produced and inserted. If a metal-based definitive prosthesis is planned, it is best constructed at this stage once the healing of any extraction sites and ridge maturation has taken place, and the coping inserted. The original acrylic resin prosthesis can then be converted to act as a spare (Figs. 3.14, 3.15).

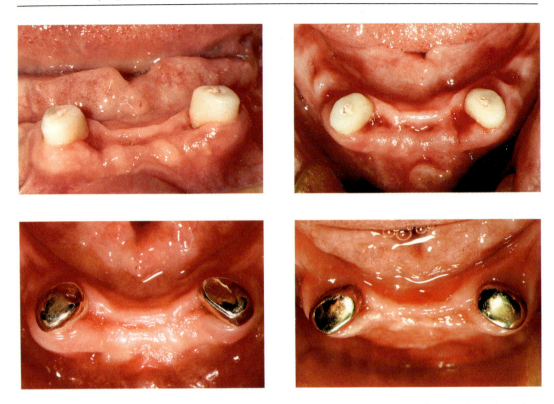

Fig. 3.14. Precious metal copings are normally constructed some 3 months after the extraction of the other teeth. A bare root face is left until this stage. If a metal based definitive restoration is to be constructed, it is made following insertion of the metal copings and the original transitional denture converted to act as a spare. (a) Initial reduction. (b) Outlined preparations. (c) Gold copings in place (3 months later). (d) 5 years later.

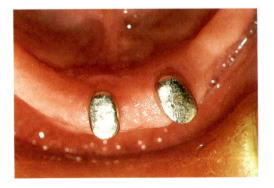

Fig. 3.15. Ten-year postoperative results of mandibular incisors. Note the patina on the metal.

Attachments

Prefabricated attachments are versatile and may provide considerable retention and stability. In some instances the additional retention available may have a dramatic effect upon the restoration. In terms of space required, attachments are normally midway between the tall thimble copings and the extremely short dome-shaped preparations that have been described (Fig. 3.16). A variety of attachments are available that range from the traditional mechanical units to those in which retention is provided by magnetic forces.

Stud attachments are particularly useful, providing both stabilisation and retention (Fig. 3.17). They may be divided into those that are extraradicular and project from a root restoration and those that are intraradicular and apply load within the root contour. Somewhat less vertical space is occupied by intraradicular stud attachments which incorporate the male component in the impression surface of the overdenture and a prefabricated component placed within the centre of the root. Bar attachments are most effective retainers and stabilisers but occupy considerable space.

Employing attachments adds to the expense of the restoration and to the complications of maintenance procedures. Attachments not only require precise location between the various components, but may place

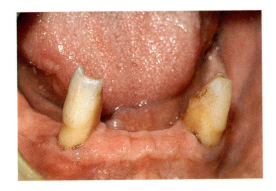

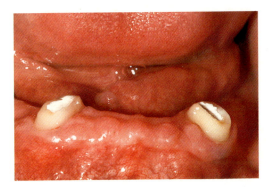

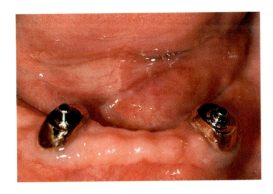

Fig. 3.16.(a) Canine teeth following root filling. (b) Initial reduction and preparation. (c) 3 months later, stud attachments in place.

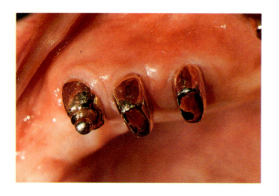

Fig. 3.17. Stud attachments are midway in space requirements between dome shaped restorations and thimble shaped copings. They can be used in conjunction with copings on other teeth.

additional forces on their retaining dowels. Nevertheless, in selected patients, the benefits provided can be most worthwhile and their popularity quite rightly continues to grow.

Root preparations for castings

Any projection above the level of the mucosa can only be accommodated by hollowing out a corresponding volume from the impression surface of the denture. In most instances, shortage of vertical space will normally require the root surfaces to be cut down to just above gingival level. Plaque control requirements dictate that the coping must not be over-contoured or bulbous in any respect. A chamfer or bevel will be required around the root preparation to allow adequate thickness of metal to support the root structure and minimise any danger of crack propagation. Overcontoured root copings and the resulting damage were frequent occurrences in the past.

Preparations for dome-shaped copings

The design of the coping will influence the preparation of the root face and the retaining dowel. Where dome-shaped copings are employed, mainly vertical loads will be applied, although resistance to lateral and rotational forces must be provided. A relatively short dowel of 4–5 mm length will normally suffice. All that is required is to provide an antirotation slot, and enough space to allow a gold thickness over the occlusal section of not less than 1.5 mm. Whether or not the occlusal contour of the dome is slightly flattened appears to make little difference in practice. A considerable amount of wear appears to take place and perforations will be found after 2 years or so if the gold coping is thin. A chamfered margin or bevelled shoulder should be used as the knife edged finish has insufficient strength.

Preparations for attachments

While the occlusal surface of the root preparation is similar to that required for a dome-shaped coping, it is important to ensure that the centre is hollowed out to provide adequate thickness of metal around the occlusal portion of the dowel. This helps provide adequate strength at the dowel/diaphragm junction while reducing the space consumption of the attachment. The anti-rotation slot also assumes an important role and the canal requires careful preparation to a depth of at least 10 mm, preferably using one of the parallel sided systems.

The dowel preparation – direct techniques

Techniques involving tapered reamers and directly waxing the dowel and coping in the mouth have been used for years and with good results. They require extensive removal of dentine and can be useful where the canal is irregularly or unusually shaped after the removal of caries. This approach cannot normally be employed with attachments unless a two-stage technique is undertaken. The apparent simplicity of the method is deceptive, as it is surprisingly difficult. Apart from the complications of reaming, preparing the occlusal surface and a direct pattern, the mechanical properties of a cast dental gold cannot be expected to match those of a wrought alloy

specially produced for the purpose. There is always the risk of the dowel's strength being reduced by contamination. Dimensional accuracy is also important, as attempting to seat an oversized dowel may split the root, whereas an undersized dowel reduces retention and allows shearing loads to be borne by the luting agent with resultant loosening of the dowel. When used with attachments, the casting should be made and tested in the root, leaving a section of the sprue as a handling aid. The casting is left unluted on the root and removed in an overall locating impression. Eventually the attachment is soldered to the abutment restoration.

Matched reamer dowel systems

A variety of differing dowels are produced by European and North American manufacturers. They are convenient to employ and give best results where a circular shaped canal can be produced in normally shaped roots. Most of the systems are designed for use with engine driven reamers so that any wobble due to a slightly worn bearing will be reflected in an enlarged canal and a poorly adapted dowel. Inaccuracies of this kind can be overcome by care with handpiece maintenance, minimising reaming speeds and, when necessary, employing specially produced chucks that allow reamers for latched-type handpieces to be

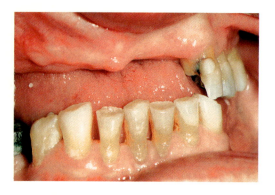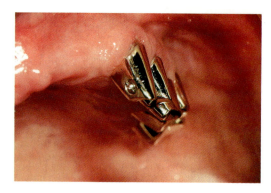

Fig. 3.18. The thimble shaped coping is useful for awkwardly distributed abutments.

turned by hand. Careful preparation of the root face and the provision of an antirotation slot are essential aspects of the procedure.

The systems available may be divided into two groups:

1. Systems in which the dowel is laboratory cast.
2. Systems in which the wrought dowel is prefabricated from a specially produced alloy.

Precious metal, stainless steel, titanium, and even carbon fibre systems are available and appear to give satisfactory results provided that a virtually parallel sided dowel of at least 10 mm is carefully produced.

The thimble shaped coping

This space consuming but versatile approach is particularly useful for awkwardly distributed abutments (Fig. 3.18). The operator is given almost unlimited scope with design which determines the stability and retention provided for the removable prosthesis. The thimble shaped copng usually forms the inner layer of a telescopic prosthesis.

Telescopic prostheses

For several decades, these most useful restorations have maintained their prominence in the prosthodontist's armamentarium. The versatility offered by this approach allows optimum utilisation of scattered or irregularly positioned natural abutments, while leaving the degree of retention and support obtained in the hands of the operator. Only prostheses requiring additional support from the mucosa and removable by the patient are considered in this text. The apparent simplicity and attraction of the approach is obvious but the thimble coping must occupy appreciable vertical and buccolingual space. Furthermore, the contours of the outer aspects of the thimble effectively determine the path of insertion of the denture. Other design requirements are the need to cover the thimble with an adequate thickness of denture base material to prevent breakages, while at the same time providing an acceptable appearance.

Space considerations normally dictate devitalisation of anterior abutments. At one time, the Miller concept (1958) was extremely popular, both in civilian and military dental health care (Fig. 3.19). This involved placing gold thimbles over vital canines and is a method that has stood the test of time, the main drawback being the bulk of the completed prosthesis. Nowadays it is appreciated that not just anterior teeth but premolar abutments as well may require devitalisation together with the occasional molar where vertical space is restricted. The retention obtained for the overdenture will vary inversely with the taper of the coping, while the adaptation of the denture base to the coping will influence stability as well. Even copings of minimal taper (approximately 5 degrees) require a height of about 4 mm if significant retention is to be provided so that careful space and alignment assessment is essential (Fig. 3.20, 3.21).

The telescopic approach still remains a most valuable restorative method. To obtain best results, the operator requires a clear idea of the

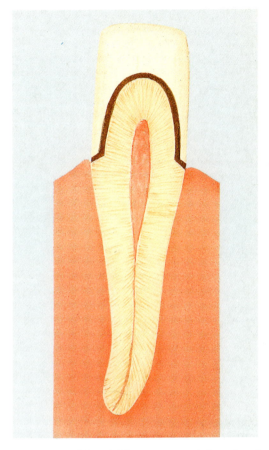

Fig. 3.19. The Miller concept involved placing gold thimbles over a vital canine. The bulk of the completed prosthesis was the main drawback.

end result before tooth preparation is begun and the use of mounted diagnostic casts is invaluable.

Preparation of the abutment teeth is a task that is all too easily underestimated. There is a common misconception that as the inner coping will be produced in the laboratory, misalignments of preparations can be accommodated at this point. This overlooks the vital aspect of bulk.

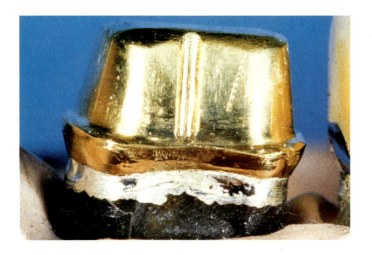

Fig. 3.20. For best retention minimum taper of the copings should be produced – less than 5 degrees if possible.

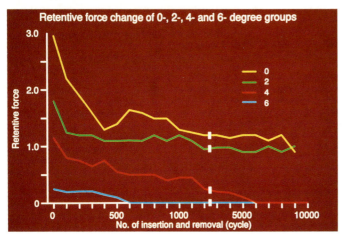

Fig. 3.21. Graph to show the effect of taper of retention (courtesy of Professor Tsuru).

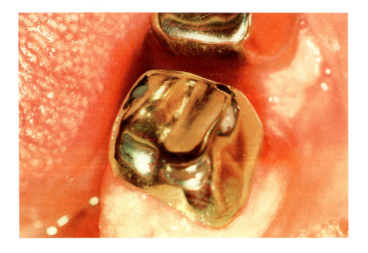

Fig. 3.22. Over a period of time, thin inner copings can become worn through.

Abutments for telescopic prostheses will be covered by two layers of metal while facial surfaces may require facings as well. All this requires extensive preparation and planning, as a poorly executed abutment preparation is one of the most common mistakes to make. The results of such errors are thin inner copings that become perforated after a period of use, together with a bulky and unsightly removable prosthesis (Fig. 3.22).

Occlusal reduction of 2–3 mm is the minimal requirement, while this type of reduction in the axial walls is more difficult to achieve. Nevertheless, inadequate abutment preparation is one of the more common errors made and leads to a bulky prosthesis or failure of castings. The problem becomes accentuated when one or more of the abutments is inclined. It can now be understood why diagnostic casts are invaluable in planning this approach. If in doubt, an alginate impression can be made of the outlined preparations. Surveying the cast of this impression will speedily illustrate further reductions or modifications required.

In surveying the master cast, the soft tissue contours need to be taken into account, as these will influence the path of insertion of the denture and, indirectly the preparation of the teeth. Although height and size of the inner coping must influence retention, the principal factor for retention appears to be its taper, assuming that the outer casting is accurately adapted.

The literature demonstrates ample evidence of the marked reduction in retention that occurs once the taper increases beyond about 6 degrees. Indeed, if the convergence angle of the axial walls is 6 degrees or less, a significant amount of retention can be provided. Unfortunately, truly parallel sided copings are difficult to produce and almost impossible for the patient to use, as finding the correct path of insertion when inserting the removable prosthesis would require a remarkable degree of tactile discrimination. If virtually parallel sides to the coping can be produced, then a chamfer is required at the occlusal edge to facilitate insertion of the removable section. The chamfer will also prevent the prosthesis jamming during efforts at re-insertion. Such mishaps are likely to speed up wear of the copings and might result in damage to the removable section as well. Generally speaking, anterior and premolar teeth will need to be devitalised to allow for the tooth reduction required, while some molar abutments can be left vital. Where extensive secondary dentine has been deposited, it may be tempting not to root fill anterior abutments: in fact, it may be virtually impossible to do so in some instances.

Support is naturally a key factor in the design. The operator is enabled to vary load distribution between teeth and mucosa by means of base extension, coping design and impression techniques. Isolated abut-

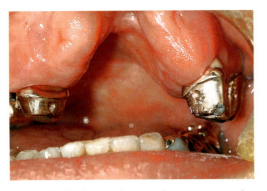

Fig. 3.23. Telescopic prostheses are valuable restorations for patients with cleft palate (15-year result).

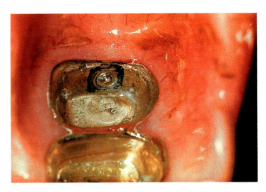

Fig. 3.24. Additional retention can be provided by a plunger type attachment.

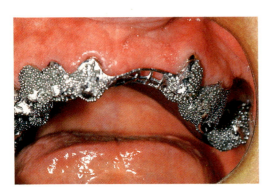

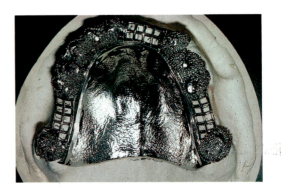

Fig. 3.25. The design of a metal major connector and its tagging requires careful thought and planning.

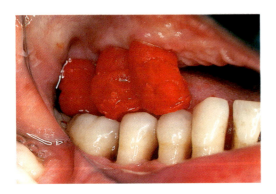

Fig. 3.26. Telescopic prostheses involve double castings. In view of the consequences of errors in jaw relations, these records should be carefully checked. Duralay copings can be employed.

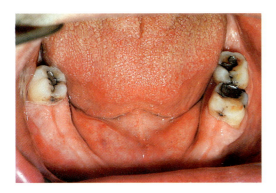

Fig. 3.26.(b)

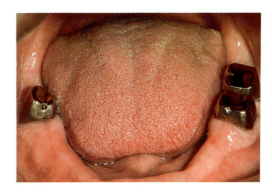

Fig. 3.26.(c)

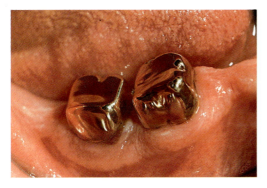

Fig. 3.26.(d)

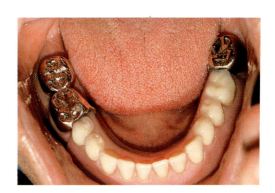

Fig. 3.26.(e)

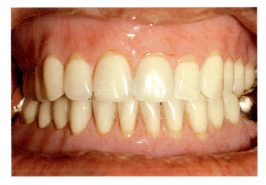

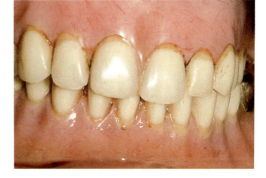

Fig. 3.27.(a) Another situation favouring telescopic restorations. (b) Fifteen years later.

ments can also be employed and, in the event of tooth loss, additions can be made to the restoration.

Jaw relation recording methods are no different from other overdentures but the consequences of error are greater, particularly if both layers of metalwork have been completed before the error is discovered.

The removable section of the prosthesis requires equal care in its planning. Since it is removable, it requires sufficient strength to withstand handling by the patient and the inevitable minor mishaps that occur. The outer crowns require connection to each other by the major connector or another rigid component. These outer crowns cannot simply be buried in acrylic resin, due to processing changes that occur.

In days gone by, there was controversy over using different metals for inner and outer layers of the crowns. The main fears were excessive wear and of galvanic action. While most technicians would agree that working with two layers of type 3 or 4 yellow gold is the ideal way to produce two perfectly adapted surfaces, it is not absolutely essential (Figs. 3.23–3.27).

Platinised gold can be used for the outer layer if porcelain is to be fused to it, although any flexing would result in cracking of the porcelain. Chrome cobalt alloy can be used; the most difficult yet important aspect is to produce well adapted surfaces. Any high spots are likely to result in wear of the underlying gold coping.

Additional retentive features such as plunger type attachments may be incorporated, but the bulk of the attachment system has to be accommodated. The prosthesis has to be designed to allow for spring changing and other maintenance requirements. For a long service life, the essential requirements of the telescopic prosthesis are to provide adequate height of vertical walls (at least 4 mm), sufficient bulk of material (never less than 0.7 mm for each casting), and a taper of around 6 degrees.

4 Screws, cantilevers, and retention systems

Overdentures must be designed to withstand a variety of different loading conditions, and it is this aspect that requires attention before the details of the individual retention units are considered. By their very nature, the retaining units are likely to be subjected to occlusal loads. This requires that the units themselves be sufficiently robust and that they are surrounded by an adequate thickness of retaining material to prevent minor breakages of the denture base around the retainer.

Small screws have been employed in dentistry for many years. Applications have included the connection of prostheses without a common path of insertion, or as retaining components for operator removable telescopic prostheses (Fig. 4.1). The screw components in these instances were not primarily load bearing units but, even so, difficulties were encountered. The head of the screw was occasionally burnished into the surrounding metal by an opposing cusp. The slot in the screw head was sometimes obliterated in a similar manner, while the restricted space available for screwdrivers, together with the ever present hazard of patient inhalation of these minute implements, was enough to discourage all but the most enthusiastic operator.

Notwithstanding these complications, those who bemoaned the difficulties of manipulation and maintenance failed to appreciate the true value of a silent ally, the periodontal ligament. The system was capable of acting as an orthodontic appliance so that minor discrepancies of adaptation between the components were overcome by progressive tightening of the screw until it remained tight. While stretching of the screw might have accounted for the initial adjustment, it is likely that few operators truly appreciated what was being achieved as the units were progressively adjusted. The advent of the load bearing implant with its comparative lack of mobility has highlighted the importance of understanding the basis of the screw clamping unit (Fig. 4.2).

Most implant systems consist of a number of components united by

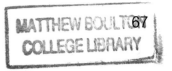

67

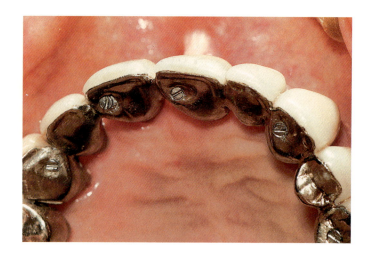

Fig. 4.1. The screw retained telescopic prosthesis has served the profession for several decades. Progressive tightening of the screw over a period of weeks could ensure the precise seating of the framework as a result of orthodontic movements. Photographed 22 years postoperatively.

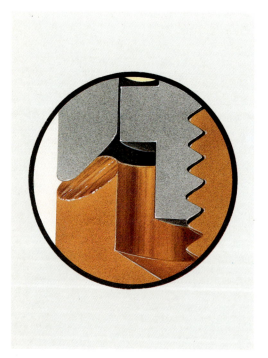

Fig. 4.2. The implant has no significant mobility, so that even minor mislocations cannot be accommodated other than by bending one of the components.

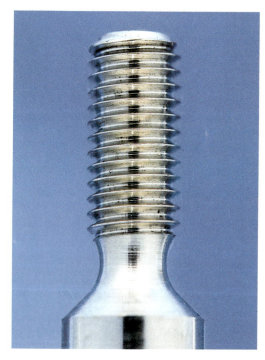

Fig. 4.3. Fundamental to the threaded fastener is the screw thread, which may be considered as an inclined plane wrapped around a cylinder.

screw threads. Many such components are also functioning as structural load carrying elements. The main advantage of using threaded screws is retrievability. The problem is that when loaded they can loosen, and unintentional loosening of screw joints is not uncommon. Fundamental to the threaded fastener is the screw thread, which may be considered as an inclined plane wrapped round a cylinder (Fig. 4.3). Before considering the mechanics in further detail, one important point should be stressed. The action of tightening the bolt compresses the component being joined and produces an elongation and resultant pre-stress in the bolt itself (Fig. 4.4). If an additional tensile load is now applied to this unit, it reduces the compressive load on the component and there is a resultant loss of clamping effect. On the other hand, additional compressive loads are of little significance.

Where overdentures are concerned, the implant components are likely to be acting as structural load carrying elements. Indeed, the potential design environments are quite broad and may involve static loading such as tension, shear or bending, or dynamic loading due to vibration or repeated impacts (Fig. 4.5). This could lead to fatigue failures in the components. The limiting mechanical property associated with these fasteners is tensile strength. A fine thread by virtue of its reduced pitch and smaller thread depth produces a higher tensile stress area to the corresponding coarse thread. In theory, if the fastening system can be given a larger preload than it is ever likely to be subjected to in service, it will always remain rigid. However, if the service load exceeds the preload it will loosen. The key here is developing the proper tensile preload in the threaded fastener system.

Unfortunately, structural joints are not always loaded in pure tension or in even pure shear. Many structural applications are subjected to bending forces which effectively result in combined tension and shear loads acting simultaneously on the fastener. There is also the problem of fatigue, and here the prime factor is the adequate preloading of the fastener to meet or exceed the anticipated dynamic or cyclical loading on the joint.

If·a threaded fastener is torqued too high, there is a danger of failure on installation by stripping the thread or breaking the bolt, or making the fastener yield excessively. If the bolt is torqued too low, a low preload will be induced in the fastener assembly possibly permitting movement which could lead to vibration. This in turn could lead to fatigue failure. The use of a calibrated torque wrench could be important and developments in this field are to be welcomed.

When a screw is tightened the preload is brought up in the stem of the screw. This tensile force acts on the screw stem from the head of the screw to the thread. The importance

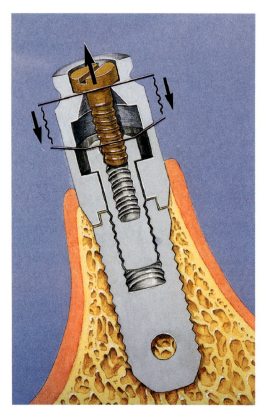

Fig. 4.4. Tightening the bolt compresses the components being joined, producing an elongation and resultant pre-stress in the bolt itself. If an additional tensile load is now applied, there is a resultant loss of clamping effect.

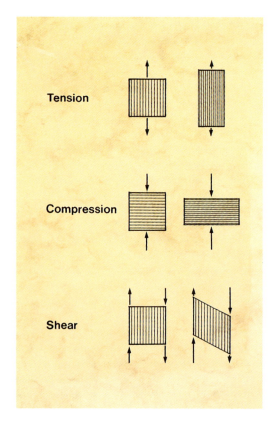

Fig. 4.5. A simplified diagram to illustrate some of the forces to which implant components will be subjected.

of this preload has been stressed because it creates a contact force between the abutment and the implant. The harder the pieces are clamped, the more stable the anchorage will be. Since all materials are elastic to some extent, the screw during engagement is subjected to tensile forces during tightening. Later on, if a load larger than the yield strength of the screw is applied, a plastic deformation of the screw results and there will be a loss of preload in the screw stem. This results in reduced contact forces between the abutment cylinder and implant, resulting in the screw joint becoming more easily loosened.

It is hard to over emphasise the importance of applying the correct torque to the abutment screw. This torque places a clamping force between the abutment and the implant. In 1995 Sakaguchi and Borgersen pointed out that, when the gold retaining screw was tightened against the gold cylinder, the clamping force on the implant increased from 118.3 to 226.4 N. The clamping forces are additive along the axis of the prosthetic components, thus the clamping force generated from tightening of the gold retaining screw was added to the clamping force between the abutment and the implant. However, the clamping force on the implant is increased at the expense of decreasing clamping force at the abutment screw abutment interface. This effect produced a decrease of 49.8% in total clamping force at the abutment screw abutment interface. This results from the tension placed on the head of the abutment screw by the gold screw within it. Now it can be understood why the abutment screw must be so carefully tightened.

Another mechanism of screw loosening occurs because no surface is completely smooth. Even a carefully machined implant surface has microscopic rough spots. As a result of this micro roughness, the two surfaces are not completely in contact. When the screw interface is subjected to external load, micro movements occur between these surfaces. Should wear of these contacting areas occur, the two surfaces will therefore come closer together. This has been termed the "settling effect" and depends on the initial surface roughness, surface hardness, together with the magnitude of the forces being applied. The rougher the surfaces and the larger the external loads, the greater will be the settling. When the total effect of this settling is greater than the elastic elongation of the screw, it works loose because there are no longer contacting forces to hold the system together. If a screw and its matching receptacle were precisely adapted, it is likely that the screw would jam as it was tightened, due to the micro roughnesses on its surface. A small tolerance is therefore normally provided, and in practice this results in the clamping loads being borne by the top two or three threads of the screw system.

It is possible that there is a significant difference in the screw stabilities of maxillary and mandibular prostheses, due to the nature of the bone surrounding the implants. The compressive strength of cortical bone may be five times that of cancellous bone, so that overloading of a maxillary prosthesis may result in more stress around the implants. Brunksi has stated that if a Nobelpharma gold screw is tightened to 10 N cm, about 300 N of preload should be generated in the component parts. Under ideal conditions he was able to obtain these figures with an experimental model. However, when a very fine dust of metal filling was placed in the joint the force obtained decreased to about 220 N. The importance of the debris-free mating surfaces, particularly around the screw head, has not always been appreciated in clinical practice.

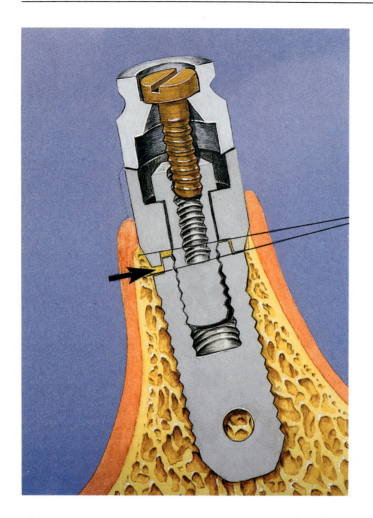

Fig. 4.6. If the abutment does not seat correctly on the implant, the gold screw will consistently loosen.

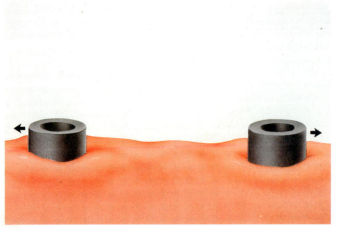

Fig. 4.7. The expansion of the stone cast can produce significant inaccuracies unless carefully controlled.

Tensile forces need not be applied directly by say, attachments, but can also be the result of leverages. These problems can be aggravated if the framework does not fit precisely on its abutment, and to achieve such adaptation is extremely difficult (Figs. 4.6 and 4.7). When machined surfaces do not seat passively and are screwed into place, threads bind. This may result in uneven thread contact, internal thread damage, increased settling, screw loosening, possible screw fracture or implant loss. Viewed from a different perspective, a great deal of the preload of the screw will have been employed in a vain attempt to unite the two components, and such an assembly is extremely vulnerable to tensile loads. This may manifest itself by continued loosening of the screw followed by a fatigue fracture.

Even the production of the master cast can produce inaccuracies, as expansion of the dental stone can produce significant imprecision unless carefully controlled. Special stones such as Gnathostone or Implant stone have expansions of only 0.02%. Apart from the importance of being well fitting, the casting must be rigid to avoid any relative motion between framework and implant under load. A large span between implants requires a connector of adequate stiffness, a point easily overlooked when vertical or faciolingual space is limited.

Cantilevers

Compared with a single unit cantilevered distal extension for a fixed prosthesis, overdentures act as a far more complex force transfer system. With the conventional fixed prosthesis, the leverage arm can be determined even if there is an element of doubt about the magnitude of the occlusal load. The occlusal load itself can be surprisingly high where overdentures are concerned, but the leverage arm is far more difficult to calculate and potentially quite large.

A factor which must be considered is the effect of leverage on the components of the distal implant abutment. Rangert and others (1991) have stressed the limitations of the strength of the edge of the abutment. With a material like titanium used in small cross-sections, this is a significant factor. It applies to the components of the Branemark system, although other similar devices are unlikely to differ significantly.

The gold cylinder and abutment of the Branemark system implant are fastened to the fixture by a gold alloy screw and abutment screw. When the screw joint is subjected to a bending moment, the pressure on the abutment side of the cantilevered abutment will increase and the pressure on the opposite side will decrease (Fig. 4.8). These changes in surface pressure and gold screw tension result in the deformation of the materials involved and the gold

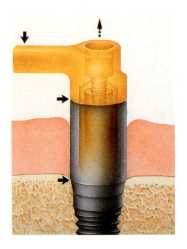

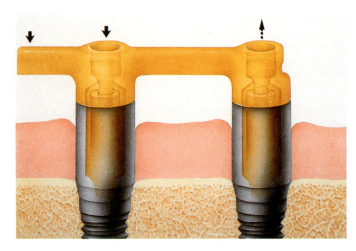

Fig. 4.8. Tensile forces may arise as a result of leverages. The strength of the materials on the edges of the gold coping abutment and abutment implant interfaces is also significant.

Fig. 4.9. Connected implant abutments alter the direction of the loads applied and the advantages are apparent.

cylinder starts to tilt relative to the abutment. The abutment, in turn, tilts relative to the fixture and this tilt registers as deflection at the end of the cantilever. As the tilt increases, the surface contact moves to the cantilever side of the abutment and the screw joint eventually opens up. Higher moments will lead to a mechanical failure – normally fracture of the gold screw (Fig. 4.9).

There is some evidence to suggest that abutment heights of 7 mm or greater may contribute to significant bending of the actual implants under load. A common example would be where a bar retained prosthesis has been used and a distal cantilevered extension is placed behind each abutment to help stabilise the pros-

thesis. In the case of a maxillary prosthesis, the additional retention is valuable to prevent the posterior border of the denture moving when even the stickiest food is chewed. On the other hand, forces applied can be appreciable and fractures of the soldered joint at the mesial end of the cantilever are relatively common and speak for themselves. Fractured screws, and even abutment screws, are by no means unknown and highlight the importance of controlling the forces applied. Sometimes overlooked is the effect of the mucosal thickness, which is also an influence on the applied forces (Figs. 4.10–4.13).

Care with jaw relation records, together with adequate base exten-

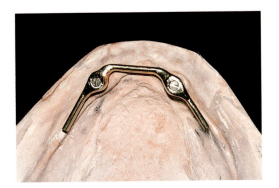 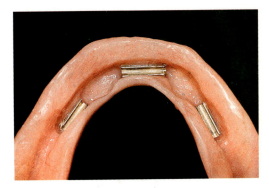

Fig. 4.10. Bilateral cantilevers on single abutments are not recommended.

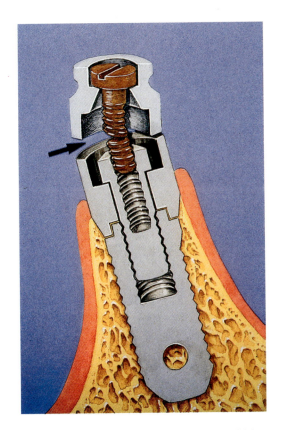

Fig. 4.11. The small gold screw should be the first structure to break if the system is overloaded – but this does not always occur.

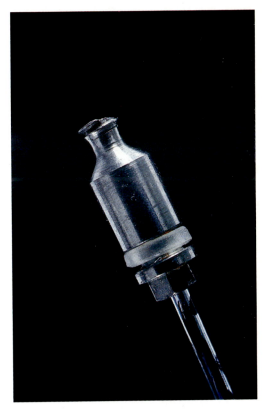

Fig. 4.12. A broken abutment screw resulting from excessive loads applied.

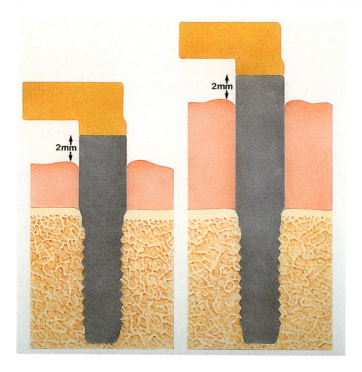

Fig. 4.13. The effect of mucosal thickness. To the observer both situations look identical, but the leverage effects on the abutment fixture interface are very different.

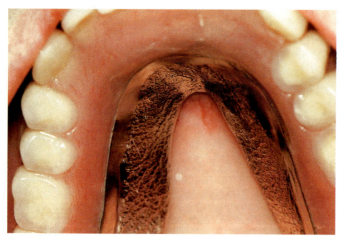

Fig. 4.14. High midline strain values dictate the use of a metal base for open palate implant prostheses.

sion, is an essential prerequisite, while the use of four abutments is considered wise practice if a distal extension bar is to be used. In these circumstances, one would expect a compression force on the distal abutment and tension on the mesial abutment. Glantz has described the overdenture as a force transfer system. The limited stiffness of acrylic resin denture bases, together with the potential leverages that can be applied, can make this force transfer system unpredictable. The stiffness of a metal denture base therefore contributes far more than strength and facilitates plaque control (Fig. 4.14).

Retention systems

Once placed in the mouth a removable prosthesis is subjected to a variety of forces in different directions. Retention can be considered as the force that resists withdrawal along the path of insertion. The ideal overdenture has inherent stability and a border seal that provides retention; the additional retaining devices serve simply an auxiliary role. Unfortunately, the ideal situation does not always apply. Anatomical considerations may dictate reduction of a flange, or an open palate design may be felt appropriate with implant supported restorations, all of which result in far higher loads upon the retaining devices.

Retaining devices may also act to provide occlusal support and stabil-

isation, irrespective of whether or not they were actually designed to withstand these forces. Indeed, virtually all retainers are required to provide occlusal support, and since there is no effective resilience in an implant system loads applied can be very considerable (Fig. 4.15). Forces applied during mastication are similar to those to which natural teeth are subjected, yet the resilience and feedback of the periodontal ligament is missing. During chewing, high loads may be applied briefly. The potential moments from loads well away from the retainers highlight the difficulty of preventing distortion of flexible tips unless some additional stabilising component is incorporated. Naturally the most important stabilising component should be the removable prosthesis itself. A denture that constantly tips and rotates around its supporting and retentive structures is likely to apply excessive loads (Fig.4.16). If the retention apparatus is strong enough, these loads will simply be transmitted further along the chain.

With our new-found exciting treatment methods, it is easy to overlook important principles. We have seen that attachments employed for such overdentures also carry occlusal loads and serve as stabilising appliances. Such functions cannot be accomplished by the flexible retaining components that must surely deform or break unless they are buttressed by a rigid structure. This must be one of the more common

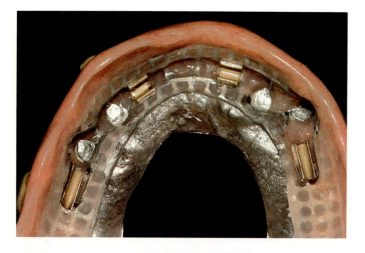

Fig. 4.15. Occlusal support and stabilisation should be provided by a rigid part of the framework. These functions cannot be carried out by flexible retentive elements.

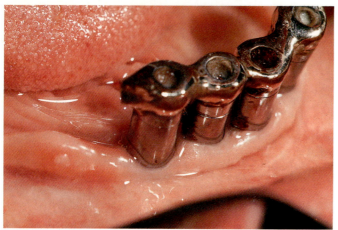

Fig. 4.16. Fractured soldered joints are not uncommon unless great care is taken.

reasons for complaints about overdentures that require continual adjustments for retention. The renaissance of bar joint attachments is due, in large measure, to their adaptability to many implant systems and it is important that their characteristics and method of application are fully understood.

Small wonder that adjustment of bar retaining clips and associated breakages are very high on the list of complications that arise with overdenture treatment. Indeed, more than one investigator has found that the frequency of these adjustments and repairs over a 5-year period outweighs the initial cost advantages of overdentures compared with fixed prostheses.

Any projection above the level of the mucosa requires a corresponding

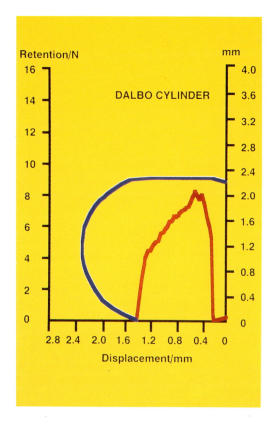

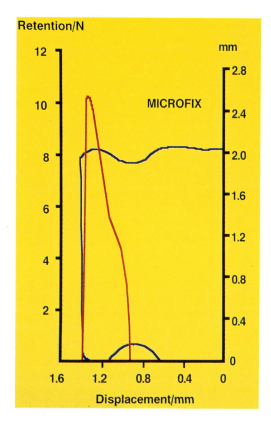

Fig. 4.17. Retention characteristics of two well tried stud attachments. The outline of the attachment, lying on its side, is in blue, the force resisting this movement, retention, is marked in red. It can be seen that a range of movement is allowed, so that retention will not slacken with the very small movements that occur in function.

hole in the denture. The bulkier the retainer the larger the hole, together with the corresponding weakening effect on the denture base. As the height of the projection increases, the faciolingual space becomes more critical, the alignment of the retaining components with each other becomes more difficult, and the correction of the path of the insertion of the overdenture is complicated. It can now be understood why there

has been a continuing search for small retaining systems. Such units would be particularly useful in the treatment of patients of Asian extraction, where vertical space is often restricted.
Preventing excessive loads, including tipping forces on the retainers, is an obvious prerequisite. However, the retention characteristics of the units need to be considered (Fig. 4.17). Take, for example, the effect of

79

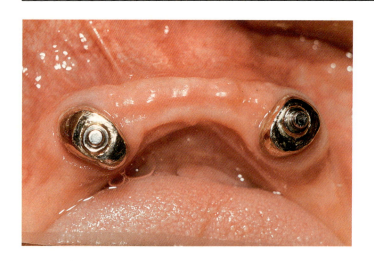

Fig. 4.18. Modern small units like the Microfix have similar retention characteristics to their larger counterparts, although they are technique sensitive.

masticatory loads upon the artificial teeth. The occlusal table will move until the displacing loads are matched by the denture supporting structures. A combination of good design and wide support should reduce this movement potential to very small levels, probably of the order of 300 microns or so, but some movement must inevitably occur. In any case, it is extremely difficult to make a removable prosthesis that fits the underlying structure exactly in the first place. There must be some discrepancy and as a result of these minor errors and a small movement of the denture base, the retaining system must work over a range (Fig. 4.18). A retaining device that provided ample retention with components separated by less than 100 microns, but whose retention fell away very rapidly so that it was ineffective at 200 microns separation, would be virtually useless in the mouth. A small retention range of

about 300 microns must be provided, and it is interesting that some of the newer smaller attachments fare just as well as their larger, older, counterparts in this respect. The older types of magnetic retainers were not particularly effective when subjected to this type of test but new developments hold promise. Once the problem of corrosion has been overcome, magnetic systems may, once again, be considered useful overdenture retainers.

Some of the larger ball and socket designs, cumbersome as they might be, provide a very wide range of retention making them less technique sensitive. Space permitting, they can be employed with implant and root supported prostheses and are straightforward to employ. Bar retainers appear to have similar retention characteristics to the larger stud systems, and are particularly useful for implant prosthodontics.

5 Stud attachments and magnets

Stud shaped attachments have served as overdenture abutments for several decades. Most are straightforward to use and possess favourable retention characteristics. Nowadays, they have applications to both root and implant supported prostheses.

Few stud attachments are entirely rigid, since their size makes it difficult to prevent a small amount of movement between the two components. Indeed, springs and other devices have been incorporated in some designs in an effort to provide a controlled degree of movement. However, bearing in mind the minute dimensions of the spring and the magnitude of the loads applied, such systems were unlikely to function as designed for more than a few weeks. For the purpose of description, stud attachments are divided into two groups:

1. Extraradicular, in which the male element projects from the root surface of the preparation or implant (Fig. 5.1).

2. Intraradicular, in which the male element forms part of the denture base and engages a specially produced depression within the root contour or implant (Fig. 5.2).

Stud devices are among the simplest of all attachments. They can provide additional stability, retention and support, while the positive lock of certain units can maintain the border seal of the denture. Mounted diagnostic casts are important aids to check the space available before an attachment is selected, as despite their minimal bulk, there are still patients for whom inadequate vertical and buccolingual space can be found (Fig. 5.3). In marginal situations, the final decision can be made after the trial insertion when precise measurements can be made. Where there is inadequate vertical space or where bone support of the roots is minimal, a short, dome-shaped coping is the recommended root preparation.

As with all overdentures, the importance of sound periodontal tissues is

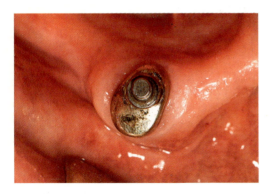 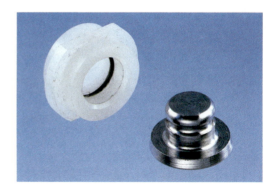

Fig. 5.1. Microfix. An example of an extraradicular stud attachment.

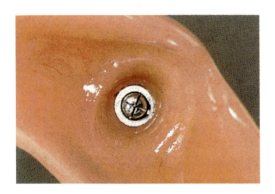 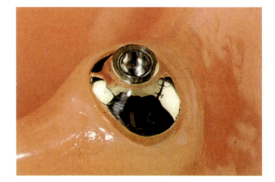

Fig. 5.2. The Ceka Revax can be used as an intraradicular unit.

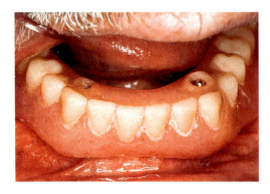 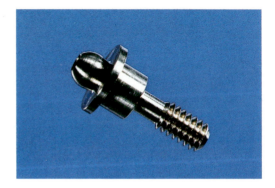

Fig. 5.3. Lack of treatment planning with mounted diagnostic casts can lead to this type of mishap. Space assessment is essential.

Fig. 5.4. Stud attachments can be employed with the Branemark and other systems, forming a substitute for the transmucosal abutments.

vital to the success of the restoration. An adequate zone of attached gingivae, together with reasonable sulcus depth, are also important requisites for a good prognosis. The stud-retained overdenture, like all overdentures, covers the gingival margins, and this potential source of irritation will be aggravated by movement of the denture base. Metal bases are easier to maintain plaque free, but the majority of stud attachments need to be buried within acrylic resin (Fig. 5.4). Meticulous plaque control and denture hygiene is essential. Failure to pay attention to these details results in irritation of the gingivae, leading to rapid downgrowth of the epithelial attachment and loss of attached gingivae. Irritation may lead to proliferation of the gingival tissues. It used to be believed that cutting a space in the acrylic resin of the denture base over these tissues was the answer to the problem. Cutting such a space merely provides a greater area into which the damaged gingival tissue can proliferate. The denture must therefore be made inherently stable and retentive, while subjected to the minimum of displacing forces. "Stress-breaking" attachments are no substitute for a correctly designed and constructed denture. A poorly constructed complete denture will move around in the mouth; a poorly constructed denture with attachments will move around the roots, leading to damage of the gingivae, periodontal breakdown and failure of the whole restoration.

Stud attachments used with implants pose problems of a similar nature. The demands of denture hygiene and plaque control remain unchanged, although the peri-implant tissues should not be confused with periodontal structures. The comparative rigidity of implants highlights the importance of denture stability. Stud attachments allow unconnected implants to be employed as denture retainers, although they can be used with connected implants as well.

Most attachment manufacturers provide excellent technical information with their products. Attachments allowing a limited degree of play between male and female units are often provided with metal spacers for use during processing. Sharp edges of acrylic resin should be removed from the impression surface, but no specific area should be cut away in this region. The important feature is that the base should be well adapted and easy to maintain plaque free.

Selection of attachments

The success of a prosthesis usually depends on careful treatment planning and attention to the prosthodontic problems; the mechanical ingenuity of the attachment is important, but must take second place. Inspection of manufacturers' catalogues will show the variety of different types of stud attachments available, but it is only possible to describe a small number. The features discussed, however, will be

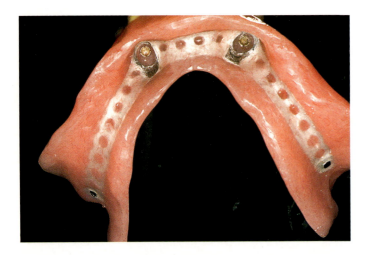

Fig. 5.5. Most stud attachments require to be buried within acrylic resin. When a metal base is employed, it will need to be designed accordingly.

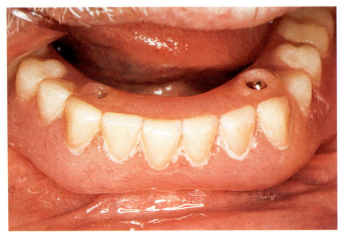

Fig. 5.6. Completing the root restorations before assessment of artificial teeth position can lead to this type of mishap.

typical of the group. The shape and size of the unit is normally the overriding consideration, although the ancillary devices that accompany the attachment must influence the choice.

The importance of correct vertical space assessment is hard to overemphasise, and it is for this reason that mounted diagnostic casts are so useful. The precise space requirements must be checked after the trial insertion stage and an occasional change of attachment may be required (Fig. 5.5). There is, however, little excuse for finding inadequate space for any attachment at this late stage (Fig. 5.6). It is this type of casual treatment planning that leads to a frantic search for the smallest attachment that can be surrounded with a minute thickness of acrylic resin. A fractured denture is the inevitable result.

Attachment movement is generally over-rated. The rigid units, due to their small size, are not entirely immovable; other categories frequently allow more movement than should ever be required.

Extraradicular stud attachments represent a large and versatile group of retainers that have enjoyed success for many years. They may be aligned with the path of insertion of the denture and are available in a variety of configurations and sizes that range from O-rings to pillar shaped projections. Retention characteristics are generally favourable, although it has come as a surprise that some of the smaller units incorporating flattened balls possess retention characteristics similar to units twice their size. Nevertheless, larger attachments are generally stronger than smaller ones and also less technique sensitive.

In selecting an attachment, it should be appreciated that space must exist for these units to be surrounded by a reasonable thickness of acrylic resin, otherwise the denture will be weakened (Fig. 5.7).

Where buccolingual space is restricted, a metal lingual connector may be employed, although the design will require to provide an adequate thickness of acrylic resin to surround the attachments. Vertical space is precious, and this valuable commodity is often wasted by inadequate or poorly executed root preparations. Additional space can be provided by osseous recontouring and mucogingival surgery, allowing the level of the attachment to be reduced. The lower the level of the attachment, the more buccolingual space there is available for the artificial teeth. Where vertical space is restricted for implant supported prostheses – and this frequently occurs in the anterior maxilla – serious consideration should be given to selecting an alternative and less space consuming retaining system such as a bar (Fig. 5.8). An individual stud retainer has to be placed over the centre of the implant which may be directly opposing the lower anterior teeth. A bar retainer can be configured to be connected to the facial aspect of the copings, corresponding with the facial aspects of the transmucosal abutments, thereby allowing the female sections, usually clips, to be placed in a more favourable position. The clips are positioned where the space is greatest (Fig. 5.9).

Intraradicular stud units have similar characteristics to extraradicular retainers, although the retentive components work in the reverse sense (Fig. 5.10). The male element forms a projection from the denture base, engaging a receptacle in the root or implant. Retention characteristics are normally satisfactory. Since the alignment is determined by the roots, any significant divergence between the roots or between the roots and path of insertion of the denture is

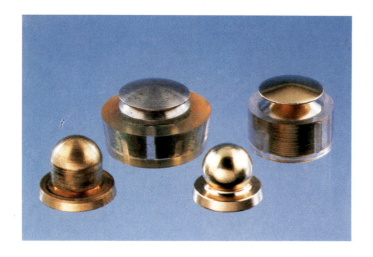

Fig. 5.7.(a). The Dalbo series of stud attachments continues to provide sterling service after nearly 3 decades of use. They are also incorporated in several implant systems.

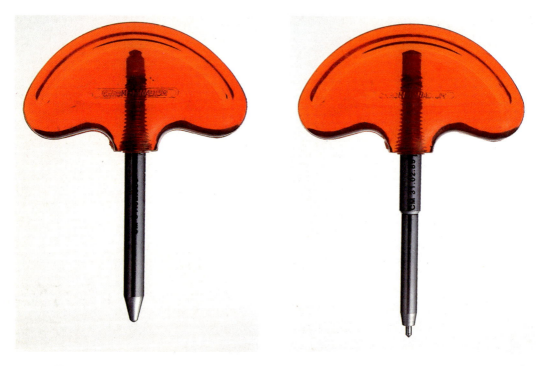

5.7(b) To reduce the retention, apply this specially produced tool. (c) Increasing retention results from careful application of force with this instrument which applies inward loads to the edges of the lamallae.

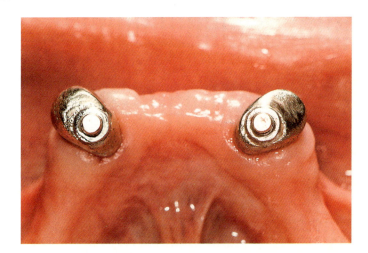

Fig. 5.8. The Microfix unit occupies minimal space and is another example of an effective retention system.

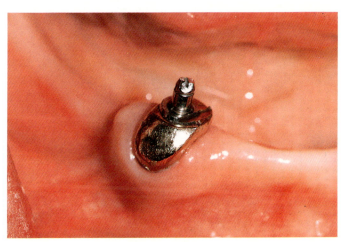

Fig. 5.9. This Gerber unit, one of the largest stud units, has provided more than 20 years of service.

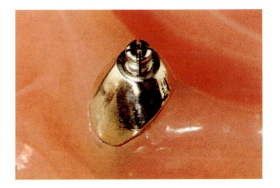
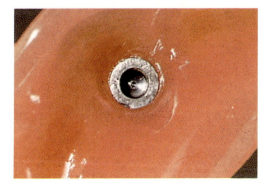

Fig. 5.10. The Ceka Revax is the latest in a series of well engineered units. In this instance the unit is employed in the conventional manner.

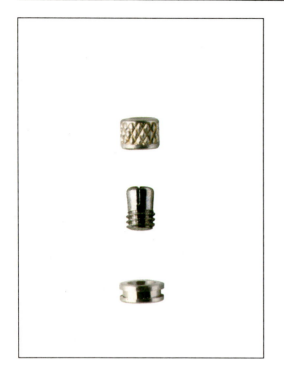

Fig. 5.11. Exploded view of the Ceka Revax extraradicular unit.

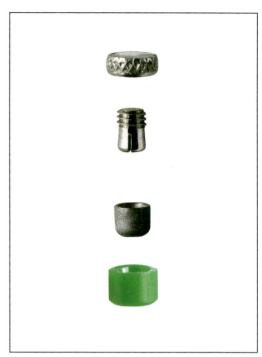

Fig. 5.12. Exploded view of the Ceka Revax employed as an intraradicular unit.

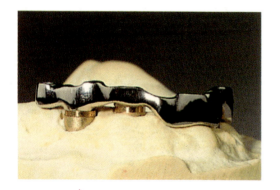

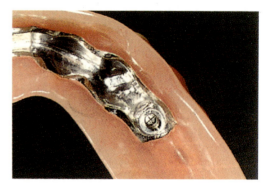

Fig. 5.13. The Revax system; can be employed in conjunction with a rigid bar stabiliser for the retention of implant supported overdentures.

likely to result in a rapid rate of wear of the male projections. These normally require replacement, as adjustments are not possible, although the replacement procedure is straightforward.

Space requirements of intraradicular units are equivalent to those of the smallest extraradicular studs. Where roots are concerned, the intraradicular units have a significant advantage in that no additional precious metal casting is required, as the preformed receptacle is placed into a hole produced by a matched reamer. On the other hand, this receptacle is likely to require extensive finishing, as it is unlikely to match the contours of the root and it does require the removal of extensive root structure (Figs. 5.11, 5.12, 5.13).

The alignment of stud attachments

Three separate considerations need to be taken into account:

1. The alignment of stud attachments with one another.
2. The alignment of stud attachments with the path of insertion of the denture.
3. The taller the attachment, the more difficult the alignment may be.

The ball and socket type of retainer still remains the most popular variety. Despite optimistic claims to the contrary, the scope for misalignment of two units is quite narrow; although divergence of about 10 degrees can usually be tolerated, excessive wear will result from wide divergencies. O-rings will also suffer unacceptable rates of wear if there are marked divergencies between the two retainers (Fig. 5.14). Intraradicular units are prone to fractures of the male elements in such situations. This is one aspect in which placing attachments into or onto the roots without the benefit of a surveyor may lead to complications. Significant divergence of roots or implants should be considered a contra-indication to this approach. Ideally, the attachments will be aligned with one another when the path of insertion of the denture is selected.

Problems of space go hand in hand with the complications of deciding the correct path of insertion for the denture (Fig. 5.15). Failure to make this alignment correctly will result in excessive reduction of the denture base and the weakness associated with it. With single implants, there is little room for manoeuvre as the stud attachment is a straight line extension of the implant (Fig. 5.16). Wide divergencies usually require an alternative approach (Fig. 5.17).

Root supported overdentures often share a common problem with the bone surrounding the remaining roots, particularly when they are canines. In some instances, altering the path of insertion of the denture may solve the problem unless there are conflicting undercuts. A typical situation would be one that arose

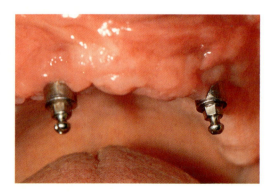 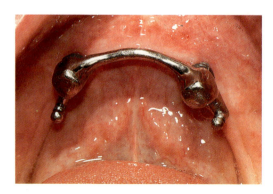

Fig. 5.14. O-rings are popular retention systems. However, changing the ring can, occasionally, be troublesome.

from anterior undercuts around prominent lower canines and bilateral posterior undercuts in the retromylohyoid fossae. A similar problem may be found in the maxillae, where the canine eminences and tuberosities produce an identical dilemma. Although surgical reduction of the tuberosities should always be considered, it may not be feasible and the problem of conflicting undercuts remains.

When all avenues have been explored and conflicting undercuts still remain, it will be necessary to reduce the buccal flange of the denture base. This is not a decision to make lightly, as the denture will be considerably weakened and the border seal lost. The lack of stiffness in the base can be overcome by using a metal denture base, while attachments can provide the additional retention. This is naturally a decision that must be made early in the treatment plan rather than as a desperate measure following the

fracture of a thinned and weakened denture. In planning the path of insertion for the metal framework, it should be spaced from roots carrying attachments to allow both for the attachment and for the bulk of the surrounding resin. The metal denture base should cover the entire surface of roots with simple copings.

The number of stud attachments

One stud attachment on each side of the arch will usually suffice; other remaining roots can be covered with simple copings. Increasing the number of attachments in a denture does not produce a corresponding improvement in retention; it may contribute to improved stability, but leads to a weaker structure and one that is more difficult to clean and maintain. Exceptions to this rule include nylon attachments, or those of similar construction, with awkward distributions of remaining roots.

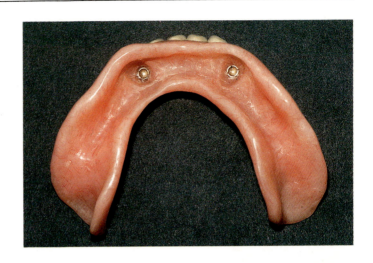

Fig. 5.15. An attachment must be surrounded with an adequate thickness of acrylic resin of at least 2–3 mm. All that projects above the mucosa represents a hole within the overdenture with corresponding weakness. Vertical space is precious.

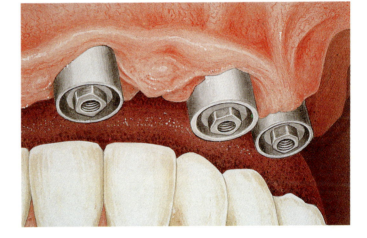

Fig. 5.16. The retention unit of a stud attachment has to be placed directly over the centre of the root or implant. This may be directly opposing an occlusal surface where space is restricted.

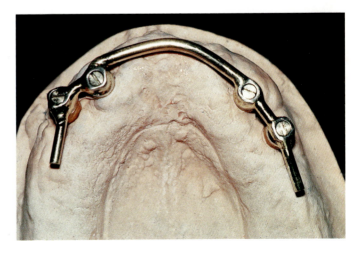

Fig. 5.17. A bar can be moved facially or lingually to the root or abutments and clips placed at the most convenient sites between the teeth. A stud retainer must form a direct extension of the implant or root.

Connecting adjacent copings

Two stud attachments on adjacent roots are seldom necessary. They would only serve to weaken the denture, complicate plaque control and produce an unnecessary level of complexity. However, connecting the copings is another matter, as rotational loads will be well resisted and inclined forces resolved in an axial direction. Space permitting, the attachment itself will need to be positioned on the strongest root, and the preparation hollowed out to accommodate the attachment with the minimum of additional bulk. The connection between the two copings will need to be planned with some care. The contours of the connecting strut must allow adequate plaque control under the base, while the strut itself must not impinge upon the base of the stud unit. An additional complication is the denture base, which must allow room for this connecting element. This type of arrangement generally works when the level of adjacent margins is about equal and there is at least 2–3 mm space between these two roots; connecting root preparations that nearly touch one another will require considerable patient skill with dental floss once the castings have been completed.

Popular attachment systems

The following is a description of the more popular types of stud units. The only inference that can be made of a system that has been omitted is simply that the author has no experience of it (Figs. 5.18–5.35).

In the past, a great deal of effort was spent in discussing the relative merits of so called rigid and non-rigid designs. Space constraints made it impossible to produce a truly rigid connection between the components, but as stud-retained overdentures are mainly supported by the mucosa, some slight movement is likely to occur. Any significant movement when impression-type loading is applied to the artificial teeth requires investigation. Such movement is likely to be the result of inadequate base extension, poor adaptation, or incorrect attachment location – factors that cannot be ignored.

Ball and socket devices, together with other attachments that allow movement, do no harm, provided the potential movement is regarded as a safety valve and not as a means of anchoring an unstable denture to a rigid root. They do, of course, possess a tendency to cause tilting forces to be applied to the roots, but that depends on the overdenture. It must be apparent, therefore, that the prognosis of the restoration is influenced more by the planning, biological and prosthodontic aspects, rather than the ingenuity of individual attachment mechanics.

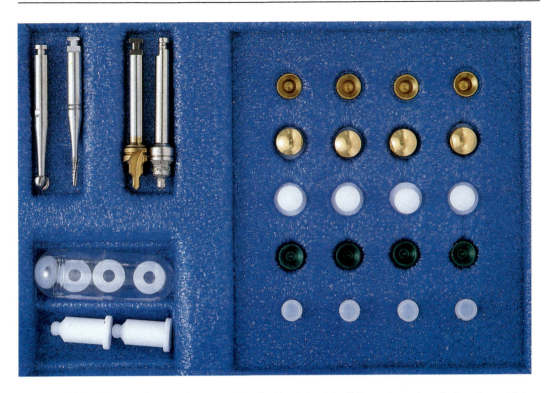

Fig. 5.18. The Zest advanced generation is the latest in this series of well developed intra-radicular units. A comprehensive kit is provided.

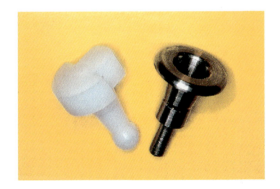

Fig. 5.19. The metal section (female) is incorporated within the root.

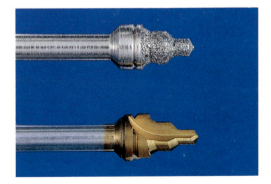

Fig. 5.20. The initial preparation may be carried out with a round head burr followed by a diamond instrument (top). The one-step procedure may be employed using the metal bur (bottom).

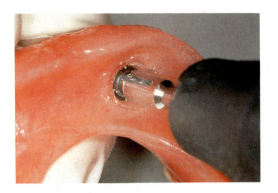
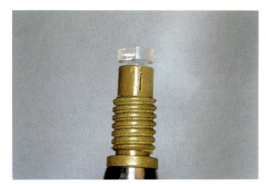

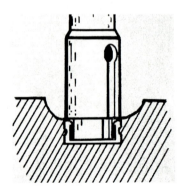
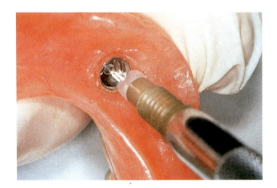

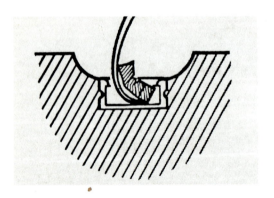
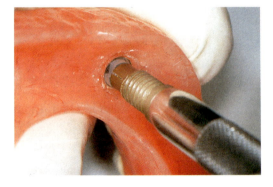

Fig. 5.21. Removal of the male unit from the impression surface of the denture is undertaken with the coring instrument. The remains of the base should be dissected with a blade or explorer.

Fig. 5.22. The replacement male is carried into place on the end of the seating instrument.

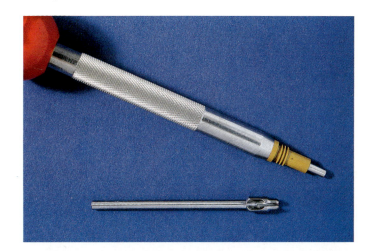

Fig. 5.23. The seating tool and cropping instrument.

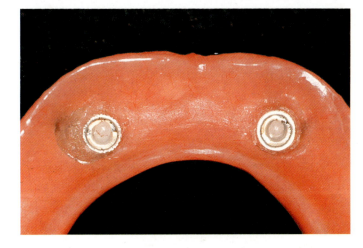

Fig. 5.24. The impression surface of the denture incorporating Zest attachments. Note the metal base for these units, which not only simplifies the replacement procedures of the male but makes relocation techniques unnecessary.

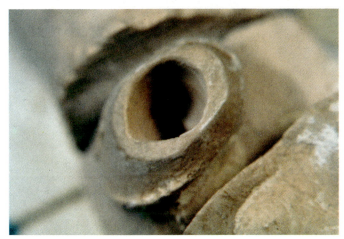

5.25. Zest units can be incorporated within gold copings. Note the extensive reduction of the internal aspect of the root that is required.

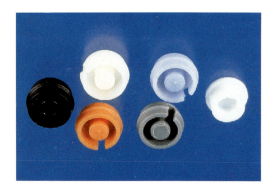

Fig. 5.26. The ERA system may be used for overdentures. Colour coded resin units provide varying degrees of retention.

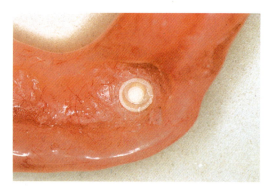

Fig. 5.27. ERA retainer within an overdenture.

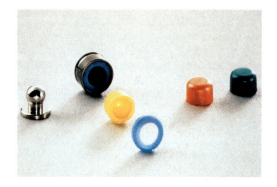

Fig. 5.28. The Pro Snap, by Metaux Precieux, is another product with replaceable retention elements providing 8, 10, or 12 Newtons. The male unit is cast on.

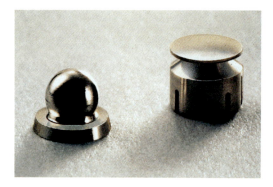

Fig. 5.29. The Pro Fix is a conventional stud retainer by the same manufacturer.

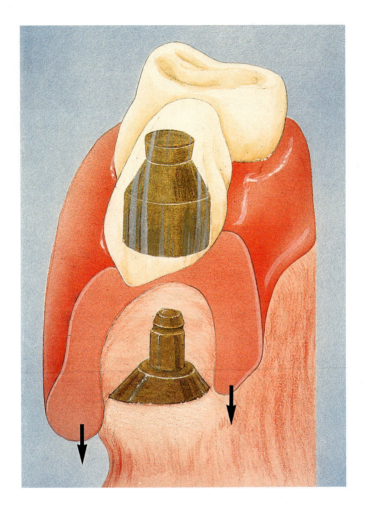

Fig. 5.30. Stud attachments work best when they are aligned with one another and the path of insertion of the denture.

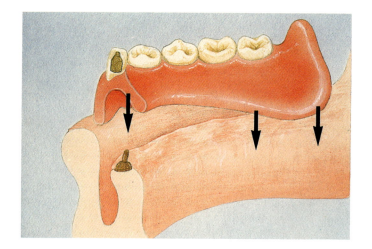

Fig. 5.31. When conflicting undercuts exist that cannot be reduced by surgical intervention, the base extension must be reduced. This will compromise both its stiffness and retention. A metal denture base with additional retention is therefore required.

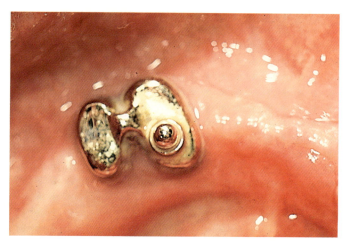

Fig. 5.32. Connecting adjacent copings complicates plaque control and overdenture construction. It does, however, result in inclined forces being resolved along the long axes of the roots. Note the lingual positioning of the stud to allow for the retroclined incisors of a Class II, Division 2 malocclusion.

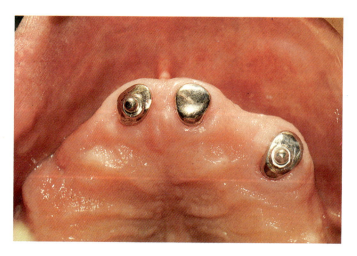

Fig. 5.33. Stud attachments can be employed in conjunction with root copings.

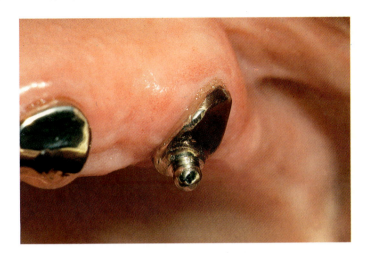

Fig. 5.34. Eight-year post-operative photograph, show-ing small amounts of wear.

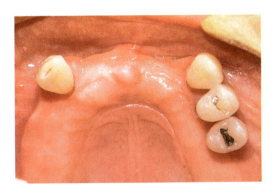

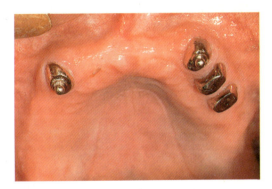

Fig. 5.35. Only one stud attachment is necessary on each side: (a) preoperative photograph; (b) Following placement of retainers and copings.

The leverage effect upon the root must be an important factor. The movements will be influenced by the design of the attachment, and also by the level at which loads are applied. The more rigid attachments usually occupy more vertical space than the ball and socket variety: dome-shaped copings occupy the mini-mum of space and leverages applied must be relatively small.

Apart from leverage aspects, a major consideration in attachment selec-tion must still be the space available for the unit, the preparation of the mouth and meticulous prosthodontic techniques. Another point to bear in mind is the availability of ancillary tools for alignment, rebasing pro-cedures, or for adjusting the retention of individual attachments.

Space becomes particularly difficult

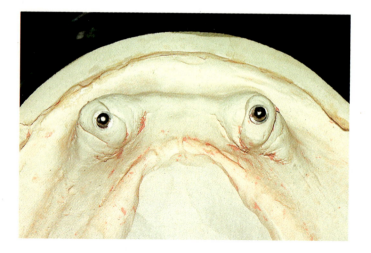

Fig. 5.36.(a) Relining, rebasing or extensive repair of a denture with an extraradicular stud retainer dictates the use of a dummy male component that is incorporated in the cast. (b) The dummy Dalbo stud retainer. (c) The dummy Microfix stud retainer.

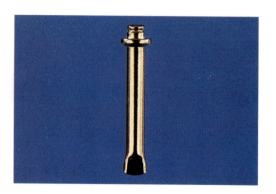

Fig. 5.36.(b)

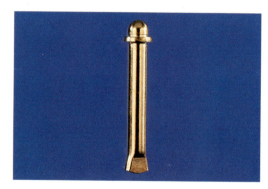

Fig. 5.36.(c)

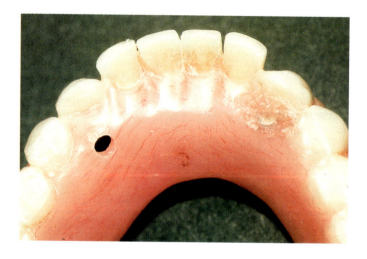

Fig. 5.37. Should it prove necessary to locate an attachment directly to the denture, always cut a vent hole. Self polymerising acrylic resin is applied through the hole.

where Class II, division 2 malocclusions need to be reproduced, as the retroclined anterior teeth encroach upon the space available. Where buccolingual space permits, attachments for lower restorations can be placed 1–2 mm lingual to their normal position.

The advent of the flattened ball design has reduced vertical space requirements at the expense of making the units more technique sensitive as the location requirements become more precise.

Since the majority of stud retainers are buried in the acrylic resin of the denture base, repairs or maintenance procedures that involve curing of acrylic resin will alter the location of the attachments due to the dimensional changes that accompany the procedure. This can be prevented by using metal dummy attachments. For extraradicular units, the dimensions represent the male component. Following the impression, these dummy units are placed within the female component before the impression is cast (Fig. 5.36). These dummies, or locating dowels, are thus incorporated in the master cast and ensure that the location of the female components is unaffected by the curing of the acrylic resin.

Relocation of an attachment is occasionally necessary. Placing the attachment in the mouth, filling the corresponding depression in the denture base with self-polymerising acrylic resin and then setting the denture in the mouth is a prescription for disaster. Always cut a small vent hole and carry out the initial location with a small amount of self-polymerising resin placed through the hole (Fig. 5.37). Minor defects can then be filled in with a later mix.

Magnetic retainers

Magnetic retention systems have been used in prosthodontics for some 60 years. Until 1970, the magnets used were made of a cobalt platinum alloy or Alnico, an alloy containing aluminium, cobalt and nickel. Both of these alloys produced disk magnets that worked quite well in paired attraction for multi-component maxillofacial prosthodontics. They demonstrated a high magnetic field strength, but their intrinsic coercivity was low. In practice, this meant that they could not be reduced in size to an extent that would allow their application for overdentures. The introduction of rare earth alloys with a high field strength and an intrinsic coercivity many times that of earlier alloys allowed the production of magnets that were not much larger than stud retainers.

The pioneering work of Gillings, at the University of Sydney, developed a split pole magnet assembly using cobalt samarium alloys (Fig. 5.38). When paired with a magnetisable alloy keeper, this produced closed-field magnetic retention. Other clinical advantages became immediately

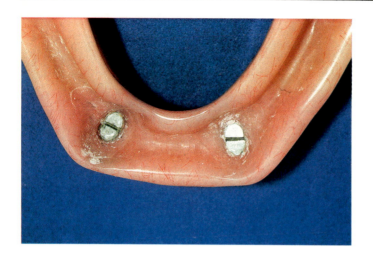

Fig. 5.38. The original Gillings magnet made possible magnetic retention systems sufficiently small for overdentures.

apparent. The magnet was placed in the denture and the flat keeper on the abutment root, so that the path of insertion of the denture was unaffected by the retainer. In fact, the prosthesis was effectively self-seating, a bonus for elderly or arthritic patients, while the denture construction was relatively straightforward. In some techniques, a spacer was placed within the denture during curing and the magnet substituted at a later stage to avoid heating the magnet. Adjustments for wear were unnecessary and maintenance should have been simpler than for mechanically based retention systems.

Initial concerns over the possible biological effects of magnetic fields were resolved, and the advantage of closed field systems over open field counterparts appeared to be one of retention characteristics. The development of a magnetisable casting alloy based on palladium, cobalt and nickel allowed a root cap and dowel to be made using conventional laboratory techniques.

The need for size reduction allied with improved retention led to the development of various sandwich type designs in which one magnet between two ferromagnetic plates effectively acted as a split pole magnet assembly, but occupied far less space.

Still further size reduction became possible with the introduction of iron neodynium boron alloys with even higher magnetic field strength and intrinsic coercivity force than cobalt samarium. The sandwich design allowed the magnet to be very slightly spaced from the keeper to accommodate a corrosion resistant sleeve. This was necessary due to the susceptibility of the magnet alloy itself to intraoral corrosion when exposed to moisture such as saliva.

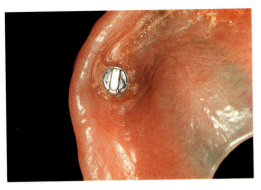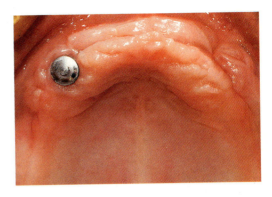

Fig. 5.39. Jackson magnet employed as a transitional overdenture retaining system on a surviving implant. The failed implant has been replaced and the magnetic unit is employed for the period of integration.

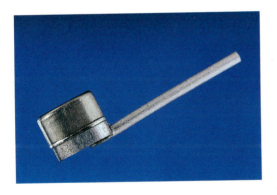

Fig. 5.40.(a)

Fig. 5.40. Two examples of the modern encapsulated magnetic retainer using the sandwich principle. (a) The Magfit 600* unit.

(b) The Innovadent (Gillings) system.

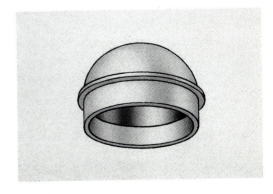

Fig. 5.40.(b)

Efforts to electro-plate magnetic surfaces, or protect them with copings, had limited success. Magnet designs which relied upon glues for corrosion protection usually failed in service. This problem continued to plague the split pole, closed field magnetic retention systems as corrosion of the magnet and the dramatic drop in retention that accompanied separation between keeper and magnetic component from functional breakaway was close to the inverse cube law. Any protection for the magnet had to be extremely thin. Greater impetus to produce magnetic retainers arose from the development of overdentures supported by implants, as it required only a small modification of existing systems to adapt them. These retainers lent themselves to awkwardly positioned, or angled implants, that would have been difficult or impossible to connect with bars. All that was required was a modified keeper to fit the transmucosal abutment or, better still, a modified transmucosal abutment that incorporated the keeper. Since magnetic retainers resist shear loads to a very small extent, some 10% of the normal retention force, the operator could be assured that only a small amount of lateral load would be transmitted by the retainer. Enthusiasm developed and several ingenious designs were marketed.

Intraoral corrosion continued to be a problem, and although encapsulated magnets were produced, initial results were far from predictable. If the capsule became worn through or damaged, the magnet could disintegrate quite rapidly. The possible toxicity of the magnet breakdown product has not been investigated, but the need to replace the magnet due to discolouration and loss of retention led to a rapid loss of confidence on the part of the profession and the pendulum of interest swung against these devices.

Despite the setbacks developments have continued using specially hardened materials, laser welding around the magnets and various forms of corrosion-resistant coatings. Hall in the UK, Gillings in Australia, and developments in Japan have produced a new family of magnets. These have still to be evaluated in practice and will need to be handled with care as the encapsulating material is unlikely to be more than 100 microns thick. The need for accurate clinical techniques remains and if they pass the test of time they will prove to be a most valuable aid in prosthodontics. Patients will need to be cautioned to remove their prosthesis if an MRI investigation is planned. For some cranial investigations it may be necessary to remove, temporarily, the magnetisable alloy keepers on the tooth roots or implants (Figs 5.39, 5.40).

6   Bar attachments

Bar attachments have been used for most of the twentieth century. They can be divided into two groups, those allowing slight movement between the components, the bar joints, and the comparatively rigid bar units. It is the bar joints that have applications for overdenture construction where two, three or possibly four teeth remain. They have also become well tried, tested and popular stabilisers and retainers for implant supported prostheses.

Early efforts at bar attachments were not always crowned with success. Carr (1988), Bennett (1904), Fossume (1906) and Goslee (1912) all published work on the subject, while Gilmore's (1913) ideas are even used today albeit with considerable modification. The swaged crowns used in those days, the failure to appreciate the significance of plaque, and the focal sepsis scare combined to hasten the demise of these restorations. Continental Europe was not so impressed with the preachings of those who blamed diseases of unknown aetiology upon the dentition and so the use of bar retention systems continued.

The bar is usually attached to the coping of root filled teeth, locking the roots together (Fig. 6.1). A common path of insertion for the retaining dowels is desirable but not essential, as the bar can be screwed down onto the coping. This method of connecting bar to coping is usually employed with implant systems (Fig. 6.2).

Advantages of bar attachments

Bar attachments lend themselves to implant prosthodontics. They act as a relatively rigid connection between implants, to which they are attached by screws. The retention characteristics are favourable and they are robust and effective retainers. Since there is a screw connection, divergence between the implants can be overcome.

When employed to connect roots, the fact that the bar is close to the alveolar bone supporting the teeth results in far less leverage on the roots than if occlusal rests had been employed. Thayer and Caputo's work (1977) suggested that the

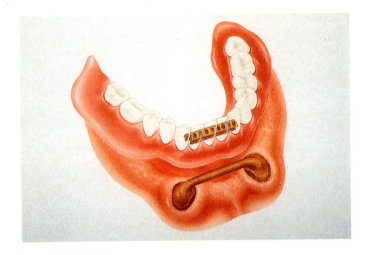

Fig. 6.1. A bar attachment connected to root filled teeth.

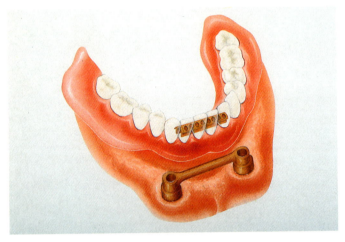

Fig. 6.2. Bar attachment connected to two Branemark implant copings. These devices are particularly useful for implant prosthodontics.

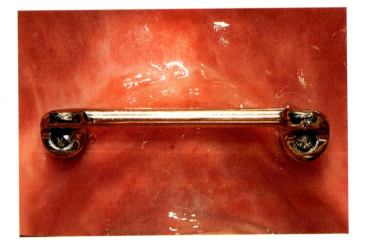

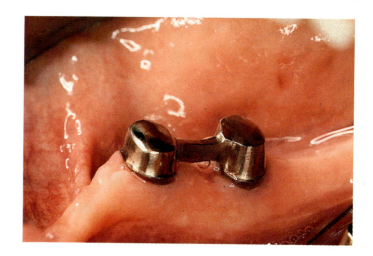

Fig. 6.3. Bar attachment used to connect a distal molar root to a more anterior abutment. It also provides a useful stabilising element for the overdenture.

joining bar resolves forces applied to the roots into a more apical direction than would be the case if the roots remained unconnected.

It is often claimed that connecting a group of teeth reduces the mobility of the unit. From a mechanical point of view, this is undoubtedly correct. The long-term biological advantages are not so clear cut, although the load sharing possibilities can only be beneficial. The design and construction of bar attachments can provide the denture with significant stability and additional retention.

There is one particular application for mutliple sleeve bar joints where their versatility is extremely useful. Following hemisection of a molar tooth, it is often desirable to connect the remaining root to an abutment anterior to it (Fig. 6.3). The bar not only allows this distal root to be connected, but can provide an extremely useful retentive and stabilising element for the overdenture.

Complications

The bulk of bar and related structures raises several problems. Vertical and buccolingual space requirements will limit applications in many instances.

Plaque accumulations around the bar must be easily removed. This complicates the design and construction of the assembly. No matter how well the prosthesis is executed, bar attachments require more plaque removal skill on the part of the patient than most other retainers. Their use cannot be recommended for arthritic patients with limited manual dexterity, nor for those whose motivation is in the least suspect.

All bar attachments require adequate and approximately equal retention for abutment retainers if cementation failures are to be avoided. The prognosis is best when mobility patterns of abutments do not reach Grade 2. Bar attachments require

considerable technical skills, together with clinical expertise. Rebasing techniques and repairs can
be complicated.

Bar joints

Bar joints allow some movement
between the two components. They
can be subdivided into two types:

1. Single sleeve bar joints (Fig. 6.4).
2. Multiple sleeve bar joints (Fig. 6.5).

Single sleeve bar joints

The Dolder bar joint is an excellent
example of this type of attachment.
This well-tried bar is produced from
wrought wire, pear-shaped in cross-
section and running just in contact
with the oral mucosa between the
abutments. An open-sided sleeve is
built into the impression surface of
the denture and engages the bar
when the denture is inserted.

Two sizes of Dolder bar joint are
produced, with heights of 3.5 mm ×
1.6 mm and 3.0 mm × 2.2 mm, res-
pectively. Apart from the artificial
teeth, a sufficient bulk of acrylic resin
must cover the sleeve to prevent
fracture, although a lingual metal
plate may be used where space is
restricted. A spacer is provided with
this bar joint to allow a degree of
movement potential. The spacer is
removed after the acrylic resin has
been cured. The retention tagging
forms part of the sleeve, ensuring
excellent adherence to the surround-

ing acrylic resin (Figs 6.6, 6.7,,6.8).
The original aim of the Dolder bar
joint design was to allow a considerable measure of both vertical movement and rotation around the long
axis of the bar. The spacer used for
the larger bar allowed over 1 mm of
vertical play – far more than should
ever be necessary for an overdenture. The bar allows some side-
to-side tilting, but lateral loads are
well resisted.

As a single sleeve bar has to run
straight, it cannot follow the anteroposterior curvature of the ridge, nor
can it be adapted to small vertical
contours. This type of bar therefore
lends itself to square arches where
the remaining roots or implants can
be joined by a straight line. Where
possible, the bar should be aligned
perpendicularly to a line bisecting the
angle between two lines drawn along
the crests of the posterior edentulous
ridges. If the roots or implants lie in a
curved arch, the space for the
denture base will be restricted lingual
to the bar and the denture may break
unless a metal lingual plate is
employed (Fig. 6.9). In some circumstances, two connecting elements
can be used to join the roots to a
straight bar, but only the straight bar
can be used for retention. However,
this is not usually an arrangement to
be recommended, in view of the
unfavourable leverages that may fall
upon the roots, descriptively known
as the "bucket-handle effect". Such
leverages falling upon an implant
may cause problems that range from

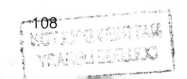

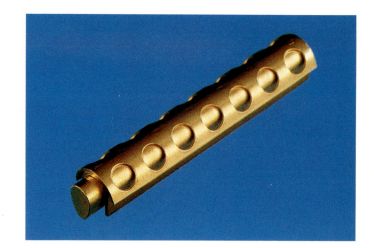

Fig. 6.4. The Dolder bar is an example of a well tried single sleeve bar.

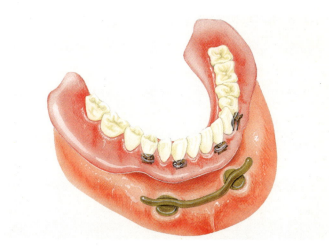

Fig. 6.5. The Gilmore, Ackermann, and derivative bars are examples of multi-sleeve systems.

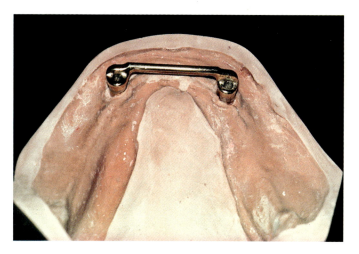

Fig. 6.6. Master cast to show position and alignment of bar.

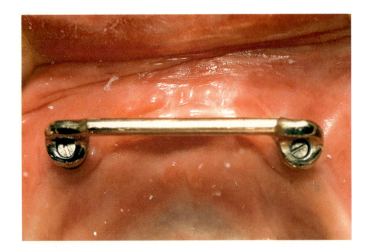

Fig. 6.7. Assembly in the mouth.

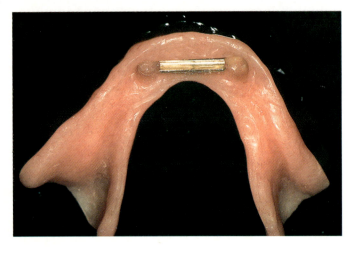

Fig. 6.8. Impression surface of the denture.

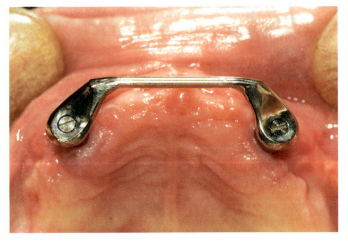

Fig. 6.9. An insufficient number of implant abutments together with non-axial loading has contributed to loss of osseointegration.

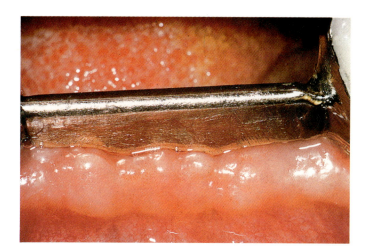

Fig. 6.10. Soldered additions to the bar scratch easily and are difficult to clean. The appearance of plaque leads to mucosal irritation.

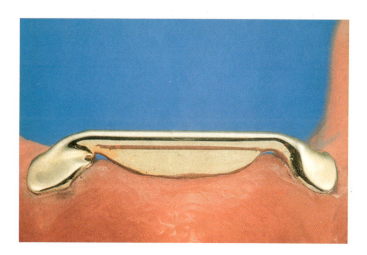

Fig. 6.11. The addition of a metal skirt simply provides additional surface for plaque accumulation.

failure of the retaining screw, or fracture of the abutment screw, to a breakdown of osseointegration of the actual implant.

Where the arch is markedly curved, the bar may occupy too much tongue space so that it is generally better to select a different attachment system. Nevertheless, there are situations where splitting the bar in the mid-line and soldering may work well. The retaining sleeve must be split into two segments. Due to the irregular shape of the mucosa, small spaces may be left under the base of the bar. Unless all the surfaces of the bar are kept plaque-free, the resulting irritation will cause these small spaces to be filled by mucosal proliferation. At one time it was an accepted procedure for the technician to adapt the bar to minor mucosal irregularities by soldered additions to the undersurface of the bar (Fig. 6.10). These soldered additions are particularly difficult to maintain plaque-free, as they are irregularly shaped and scratch easily. Again, the result is irritation.

Another method that has been tried is to employ a modified bar that includes a skirt. Unfortunately, this skirt simply provides additional surface area for plaque accumulation (Fig. 6.11).

Where there are marked irregularities of the mucosa and mucogingival areas, preliminary minor surgery usually gives the best results. A thin wedge of tissue is removed from the area to be covered, thereby taking more away from the high areas than from the low ones. This technique not only provides for better adaptation, but usually contributes more space for the attachment unit. Where intermaxillary space is restricted and bone contours are generous, bone reduction can provide most helpful additional space. This can be particularly useful when used in conjunction with implants.

Where a large depression is found, the bar can be cranked into it with two connecting elements, thereby reducing the space it occupies. Plaque control would be simplified by providing a large cleansable space of more than 4 mm between bar and mucosa. Unfortunately, there is seldom adequate space for this arrangement unless across a cleft palate or an area of gross resorption. For the majority of patients the bar needs to be placed in even contact with the mucosa.

Space problems have been stressed for all types of bar retainer, and space is a particularly precious commodity in the lower anterior region. Space is required for the bar and sleeve, a thickness of acrylic resin and for the artificial teeth. Placing the bar slightly lingual to the crest of the edentulous ridge may help make room for the necks of the lower teeth. However, the reduced lingual thickness may weaken the denture and a metal lingual plate will be necessary.

One of the more common mistakes associated with bar-joint prostheses arises when an inexperienced operator attempts to push out the necks of the lower anterior teeth in an effort to make room for the bar. This gives the patient an unpleasant appearance, as though with a swollen lip and a mouth perpetually full of food. Appearance apart, the lip will exert a displacing action on the denture.

Dolder's early work showed that the space between the sleeve and bar was quickly lost, probably as a result of resorbtion of the edentulous ridge. Rather than relocate the sleeve at this stage, a more satisfactory approach is to rebase the denture with the spacer inserted. After all, it is loss of support to the impression surface of the denture that has resulted in this subsidence. However, when this impression is made, no load should be applied distal to the bar, for this might cause the denture to rotate around the bar. The rebasing procedure will have altered the relationship of the occlusal surfaces to the

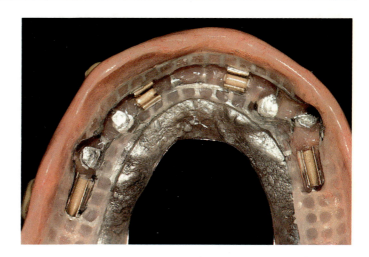

Fig. 6.12. Impression surface of an implant retained overdenture. Note the occlusal stops that have been provided.

mucosa and a check record will be required.

Quite apart from damage caused to the mucosa and edentulous ridge, it is obviously unsatisfactory to construct a denture that requires frequent rebasing or relocating procedures in the mouth. As with all other prostheses, the main object must be to gain support from the maximum possible area and reduce to a minimum any displacing loads falling on the denture. When used for retaining overdentures, the principles of complete denture construction must take precedence over mechanical considerations of attachments. The main object must be to gain maximal support and reduce displacing forces to a minimum.

Despite the potential for movement, the manner in which the denture has been constructed should make it unnecessary to cut away areas of the impression surface around the gingi-

val margins. The removal of sharp edges is, of course, another matter. A denture that moves perceptibly in the mouth requires attention. It may require rebasing, a relocating procedure, or remaking, but if a continuous movement is allowed to take place unchecked it will cause damage to the denture-supporting structures.

The high incidence of maintenance complications with implant supported overdentures has been discussed in an earlier chapter. The leverage potential when cantilevers are employed is surprisingly large, as the loads applied to the system are considerable. It is normally considered wise practice to incorporate an occlusal stop in the design (Fig. 6.12).

So far, the bar has been described as if it were positioned approximately at right-angles to the sagittal plane. This is the position in which it works best. However, Dolder has suggested that his bar be used where there are just two teeth or roots on the same side, such as a canine and first molar. In this case, the bar joins the two roots and runs along the crest of the ridge. Any rotation is sideways.

Single sleeve bars may be waxed and cast in one's own laboratory. The dimensions of the bar must exceed those of a specially manufactured attachment and the complications are considerable. The thickness of the bar cannot be less than 2 mm if a well-fitting sleeve is to be produced as well.

A bar joint that has become popular in the USA is known as the Baker clip. It is available in a no. 12 or 14 gauge bar size. The sleeve requires roughening to provide retention for the acrylic resin as, rather like the earlier Dolder bar joints, no retention tags are provided. The sleeve can be sectioned if the bar is not run in a straight line.

Multiple sleeve joints

The retaining sleeves, or clips as they are sometimes known, are relatively short. This allows the bar to follow the curvature of the ridge as well as to be adapted to its vertical contours. The versatility allowed by this approach is considerable and it has become popular with implant supported overdentures. In the anterior maxilla this method is often employed with a curved arch. However, the leverage potential should be appreciated. Sleeves can be

placed at sites with the greatest amount of space.

The history of multiple sleeve bar joints extends back to at least 1913, when Gilmore proposed a retainer of this type. Ackermann and other workers have made modifications that are widely used today. In selecting the profile of the bar, the length of the span must be taken into account, as the connection between the abutments must be rigid. Failure to achieve this rigidity can lead to stress concentrations around implants and endanger their integration within the bone (Fig. 6.13).

Of the various cross-sections available, the circular section is the most versatile as it can be bent in all planes. Pear-shaped and oval cross sections are available. Wax and plastic patterns are also produced. These are cut and adapted before casting, a procedure that requires a great deal of attention to detail.

When more than one sleeve is incorporated in an anteroposterior curve, it is likely to prevent hinge rotation. This is normally of little clinical significance if the denture base is well adapted and correctly extended. Problems often arise with implant supported maxillary dentures with an open palate design, where a stabilising component has been omitted. Multiple sleeve systems lend themselves to distal cantilevered extensions, as the small sleeves allow for an extension of less than 7 mm to provide retention. The use of cantilevered extensions nor-

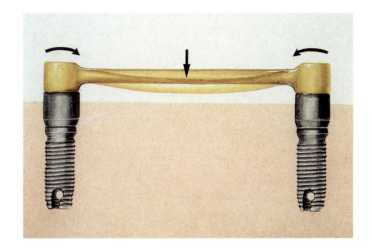

Fig. 6.13. Failure to produce a rigid connection can lead to stress concentrations around the implant and endanger their integration.

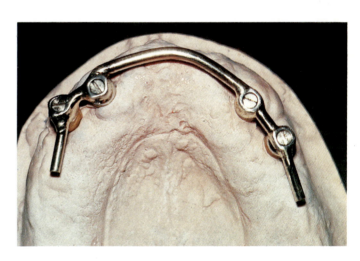

Fig. 6.14. The use of cantilevered extensions requires at least four implant abutments. Sleeves positioned on the extension will prevent any tendency for the distal part of the maxillary denture to drop.

mally requires at least four implants. Sleeves positioned on the extension will prevent any tendency for the distal part of a lower denture to rise when sticky foods are chewed. In the maxilla this becomes even more important, ensuring that there is no tendency for the posterior border of the upper prosthesis to drop (Fig. 6.14).

The relatively small sleeves of these retaining systems could be subjec-ted to considerable forces. Occlusal stops and stabilising components should always be incorporated in the design of contact adjustments and occasional breakages are to be avoided. Metal sleeves are secured within the acrylic resin by retention tags.

Of the various sleeves produced, two designs of tagging should be con-sidered. The tagging must be at right angles to the bar, or parallel with it.

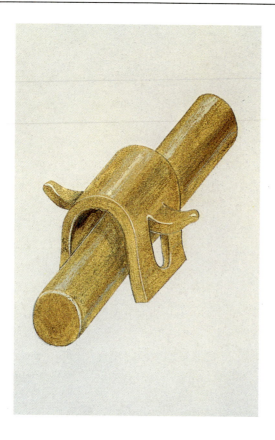

Fig. 6.15(a) The sleeves of the Ackermann bar are examples of those with retention tags that project buccolingually.

(b) However, clips featuring two designs of retention tags are now available for the Ackermann bar. These clips can also be employed with the Hader bar or other bars with a 1.8mm diameter.

Fig. 6.15.(a)

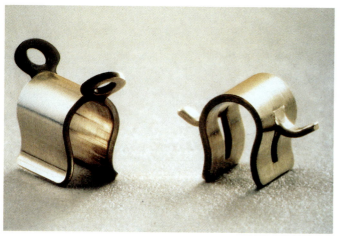

Fig. 6.15.(b)

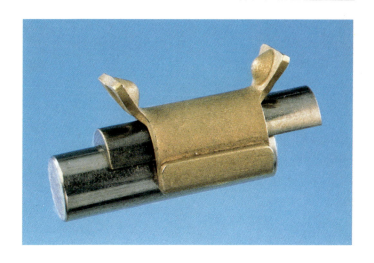

Fig. 6.16.(a) The C.M. bar retention tags project in the long axis of the bar. (b) The retention tag with a hole punched through has been found to be somewhat more fracture resistant – the reverse of what one might expect.

Tagging at right angles to the bar is well adapted to resist rotational forces applied to the sleeve (Fig. 6.15). On the other hand, the tagging encroaches still further on bucco-lingual space requirements and this produces more complications with the arrangement of the artificial teeth. Furthermore, during relocation procedures it is difficult to cut such a sleeve away from the denture without damaging the tagging or the artificial teeth. Tagging parallel with the bar simplifies both relocation procedures and arrangement of artificial teeth. The drawback is that the tagging must encroach upon vertical space in order to provide the necessary side-to-side resistance required. The sleeves may not resist rotational forces quite as well as those retained by right-angle tags, although it must be understood that significant rotational forces imply a poorly designed or constructed denture.

The sleeves of the Ackermann bar are examples of those with tags that project buccolingually. The CM bar is similar in profile to the circular Ackermann bar. The diameter is 1.9 mm and the similarity is close so that the CM sleeve can be used on the Ackermann bar. The CM bar is produced in precious and semi-precious alloys, the latter recommended for long spans. The retention tags of the sleeve project in the long axis of the bar and this simplies relocating procedures, if required (Fig. 6.16). Two types of sleeve are manufactured; the most popular has short flanges that do not project below the base of the bar. The longer flanges are employed where the bar has to be bent in the vertical plane over a short distance. The CM type of bar with the smaller sleeves has established itself as a firm favourite for use with implant supported maxillary overdentures.

117

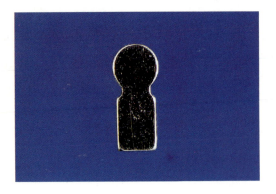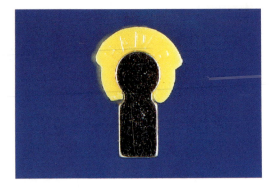

Fig. 6.17. The Hader bar incorporates a resin sleeve that is speedily replaced when it slackens. Another notable feature is that the sleeve seats directly on the bar with no intervening spacer.

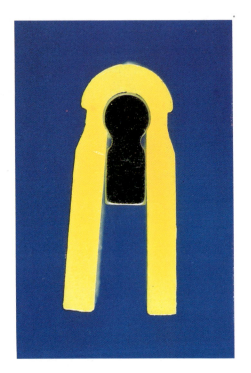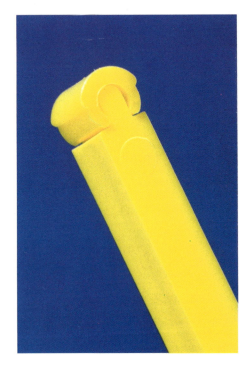

Fig. 6.18. The manufacturers provide a special space maintaining device that is placed in the wax-up of the denture base. It ensures that the denture base is properly contoured to accept the retaining sleeve.

Fig. 6.19. A special handling device is produced for the sleeve.

The Hader bar joint is now well established as a retainer for both root supported and implant supported prostheses (Fig. 6.17). The manufacturers provide prefabricated plastic patterns that are adapted on the master cast and then cast in the alloy of choice (Figs 6.18, 6.19). As with other plastic forms, this allows considerable scope for manoeuvre in adaptation of the bar to the edentulous ridge. It is the sleeve of the Hader system that sets it apart from the others (Figs 6.16–6.19) as this is also produced in plastic. An ingenious design allows speedy replacement of the sleeves when their retention has slackened, as they cannot be adjusted. However, the replacement of the sleeves is a relatively rare occurrence. Another notable feature of the sleeve is that it seats directly on the bar with no intervening spacer. As a result, it provides support as well as retention. It is also possible to substitute metal sleeves of the CM bar as the dimensions are similar.

Bar attachments on implants

Jemt has shown that the bar supporting and retaining maxillary overdentures on implants plays a significant role in its efficiency. Increased occlusal force capacity with the bar and clip suggested that these components withstood an appreciable load. Indeed, when fixed prostheses were substituted, the maximum occlusal force hardly changed in the short term, although it did increase over a period of time. The study further indicated that the velocity of the opening phase of the mandibular movement was related to the stability of the restoration placed in the mouth, a factor that will influence masticatory efficiency.

Although the principals of root and implant supported bars are similar, there are important differences. The implant has no periodontal ligament to accommodate minor discrepancies of adaptation and the implant is unlikely to be placed in a site corresponding with the position of the root it replaces. Indeed, the pattern of resorption of the maxilla may result in the implant being some 7–10 mm palatal to the root position (Fig. 6.20). Complications that may arise include the distortion of the shape of the anterior palate unless the bar is attached to the facial surfaces of the implant copings. Vertical space available for the copings may be less than expected if the implants are directly opposite the lower anterior teeth. One of the advantages of the bar assembly is the ability to place the retaining clips where there is the greatest space, and to provide short cantilevers when sufficient abutments are available. The stabilising effect of a short (7 mm) maxillary cantilever and retainer is quite remarkable but should only be used in conjunction with four abutments (Fig. 6.21). Although the use of angled abutments is far from ideal, where they have to be employ-

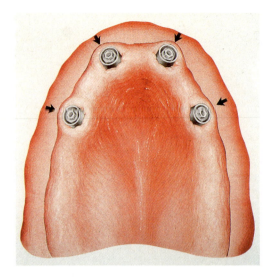
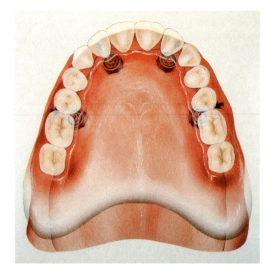
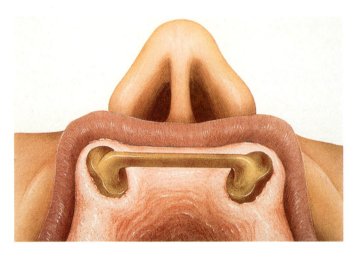

Fig. 6.20.(a) and (b) Maxillary resorption may result in the implants being placed some 7-10mm palatal to the root position. (c) Compare the canine eminence and root position where teeth remain.

ed the bar connection does, at least, minimise the effects of non-axial loading (Figs 6.22, 6.23).

Bar attachments are normally more straightforward to employ on implant supported mandibular dentures. Any distal cantilever opposing maxillary teeth will need to be strengthened, in view of the significant loads that may be applied. Once again, four abutments are normally required before a cantilever can be considered. Minor faciolingual malpositioning of implants can be accommodated by suitable positioning of the bar.

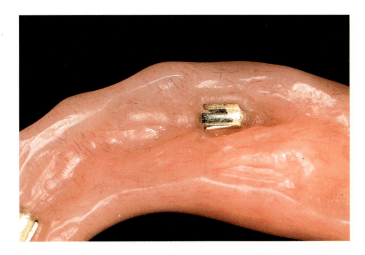

Fig. 6.21. The stabilising effect and added retention of a small clip on a short cantilever is quite remarkable. However, at least four abutments are required for this approach.

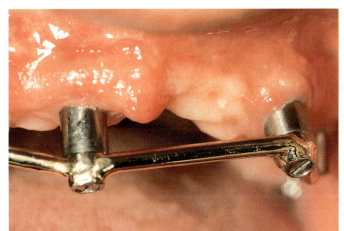

Fig. 6.22. Standard abutments can be employed when implants are only moderately misaligned.

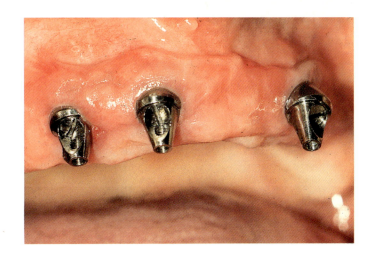

Fig. 6.23. Angled abutments are far from ideal but connecting them minimises the effects of non axial loads.

Technical considerations

Insufficient space for the attachment is a common problem. While hardly technical, it is a problem that may first become apparent in the laboratory. Measurement of vertical and bucco-lingual space should have been part of the preliminary treatment, but carelessness at this early stage may become obvious comparatively late in the therapy when the bar is set up on the master cast after the final trial insertion.

The wax-up of the trial insertion is conventional, and when the position of the anterior artificial teeth has been decided, it is then recorded with a silicone mask (Fig. 6.24). This mask allows the teeth to be removed and subsequently replaced in exactly the same position (Figs 6.25, 6.26).

If, at this late stage, insufficient room is available, a smaller bar attachment will have to be selected. The multi-sleeve bar joints are useful. Where the space problems do not allow this approach, the treatment plan may need to be reviewed, as raising the level of the occlusal plane, or pushing forward the necks of the anterior teeth as last-minute attempts to position the attachment, seldom succeed. They result in prosthodontic problems of even greater magnitude that often require the remaking of the entire restoration. Like most other attachments, bar joints dictate the use of acrylic resin artificial teeth due to space considerations.

Although careful treatment planning should prevent malaligned implants, such placements do occur and, occasionally, are not discovered until a late stage in therapy. It is here that angled abutments may be considered (Figs 6.27–6.29).

Spacers are provided with most bar joint systems to ensure that a small gap is preserved between the sleeves and bar during processing. The spacer is then removed. The Dolder bar joint spacers are generally too large. It is usually more convenient to employ the spacer for the smaller bar when the larger bar is used; when the smaller bar is employed the spacer is thinned slightly.

The free edges of the sleeve should be just clear of acrylic resin to enable them to have a slight clip action, but the amount of relief required is small. If a large relief is allowed, it creates a space when the denture is in position.

Adjustments for retention must be carried out with care (Fig. 6.30). They normally involve minute distortions of the free end of the sleeve, using a dental instrument for the purpose. While straightforward for small, single sleeve bars, the longer sleeve of the Dolder bar is more difficult to adjust in this manner. The manufacturers have therefore produced special instruments that may be used to deform the edge of the sleeve to increase retention. Particularly useful devices are also produced to reduce retention, should this have been inadvertently overtightened Figs 6.31, 6.32).

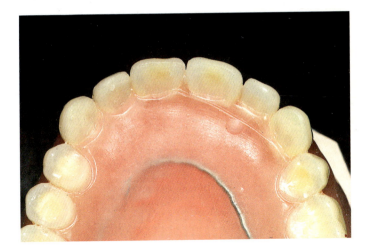

Fig. 6.24. The position of the artificial teeth should be decided with a trial insertion before the metalwork is constructed.

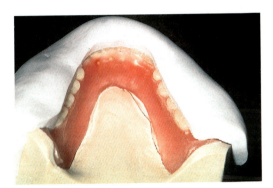
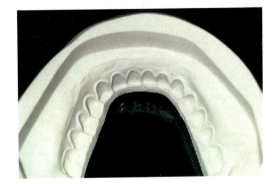

Fig. 6.25. A silicone mask is used to record the position of the teeth for a mandibular prosthesis.

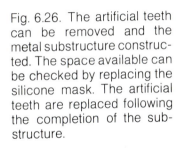

Fig. 6.26. The artificial teeth can be removed and the metal substructure constructed. The space available can be checked by replacing the silicone mask. The artificial teeth are replaced following the completion of the substructure.

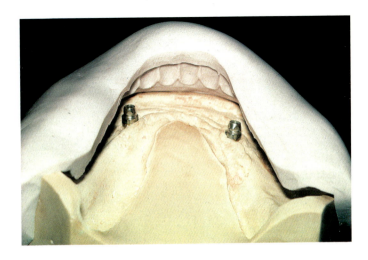

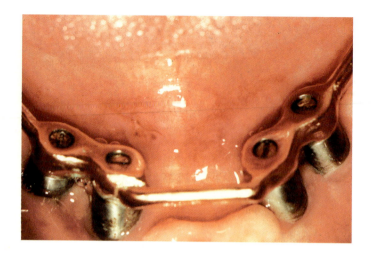

Fig. 6.27. Lingual inclination of the implants causing tongue cramping. Inserting the overdenture compounds the problem.

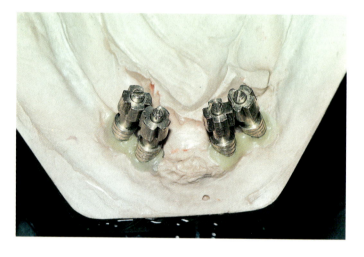

Fig. 6.28. New master cast produced with four single tooth copings. The angulation can be clearly seen.

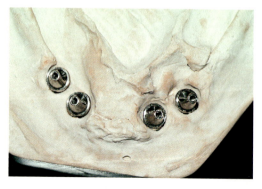
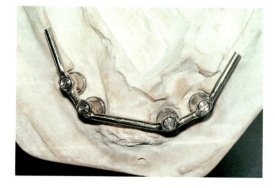

Fig. 6.29. Angled abutments allow the superstructure to be positioned facially and an acceptable removable prosthesis can now be constructed.

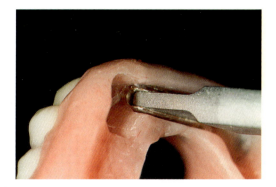
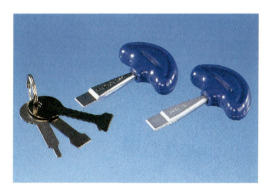
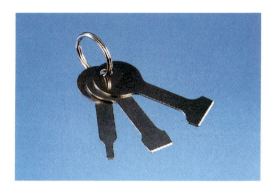
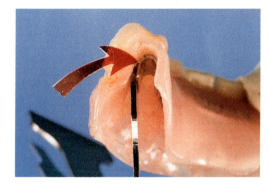

Fig. 6.30. Adjustments for retention must be carried out with care using the special instrument when available. The blue devices slacken the retention of the Dolder bar and are used prior to initial insertion or if the sleeve has become accidentally distorted in use. The small keys are employed to increase retention.

Fig. 6.31. The space under the bar has been blocked out prior to the impression. This blocking out procedure is also employed when a sleeve is to be relocated in the mouth. It is essential to ensure that no self-polymerising resin can flow under the bar.

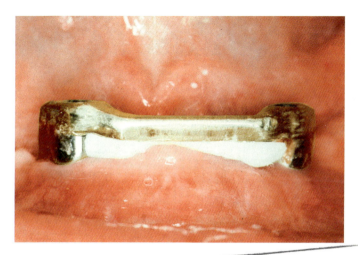

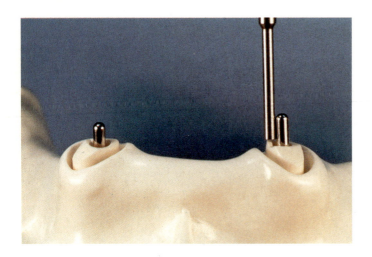

Fig. 6.32. Determine the path of insertion and check the parallelism of the root canal posts.

Prefabricated bars, like the Dolder bar, may be cranked to adapt to certain vertical contours of the ridge. A small connecting section can also be employed to approximate it to anteroposterior curvatures of the ridge, but the dangers of using other than small connections have already been mentioned.

A section of bar, longer than the edentulous space, is softened by heating to dull red and plunging in water. A V-shaped cut is made into the bar and the cut closed by bending the bar. The joint is then fluxed and joined with a high fusing solder. After soldering, the bar should be annealed before further adaptation is attempted.

Since the overdenture is acting as a force transfer system, it is apparent that loads applied from the removable prosthesis to the bar will, in turn, be transmitted to the solder joint. Failures of these joints under load are by no means uncommon and the process of soldering requires care and skill. The clinician should be aware of the problem involved (Figs. 6.33-41). Multisleeve bars are usually easier to adapt to the master cast, although annealing will be required. Both single and multisleeve bars will need to be soldered to the abutment crowns. The soldering of any bar prosthesis requires a great deal of expertise and care, particularly when a wrought bar is to be joined to a highly platinised gold crown. No matter what alloy is employed, some distortion can easily arise and the effect of a comparatively small distortion is greatly magnified when the span of the prosthesis is long and may give rise to a pronounced rock on the master cast. All sections need to be annealed (usually 5 minutes at 70°C) before assembly for soldering. After soldering, full heat hardening treatment is necessary.

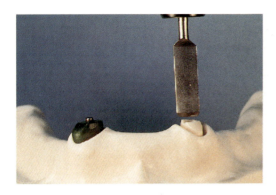 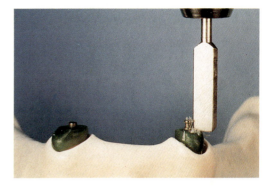

Fig. 6.33. Prior to waxing the root caps, determine the occlusal thickness of the wax and model the root caps at right angles to the path of insertion using the wax knife.

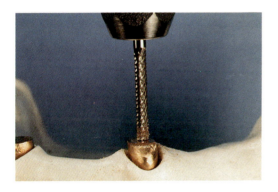 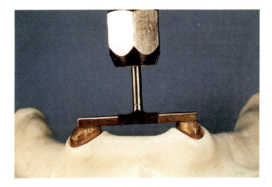

Fig. 6.34. After casting and fitting the root caps, determine the final occlusal thickness and mill the root caps at right angles to the path of insertion.

Fig. 6.35. Position the bar in the correct relation to the roots and edentulous ridge. Then align it with the path of insertion using the special connector for the surveyor.

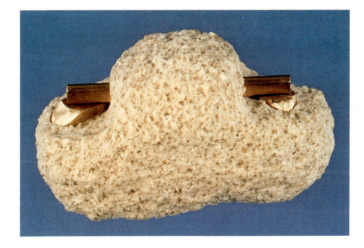

Fig. 6.36. Invest with soldering investment, leaving the soldering area free to give good access for the flame.

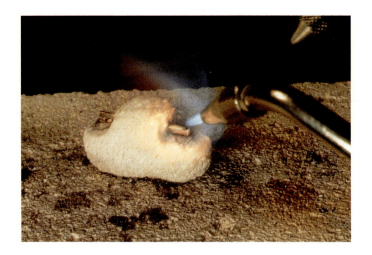

Fig. 6.37. Prior to soldering, be sure that the liquidus of the solder corresponds with that of the casting alloy, then apply flux to the root caps. Warm up the soldering block with the flame to the liquidus temperature of the solder (red colour). When the soldering block has reached the working temperature, keep the flame on one side of the bar while applying the solder to the other. The solder will readily flow underneath the bar because the solder always flows to the warmest point.

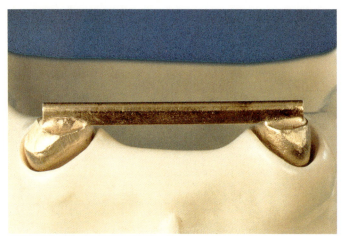

Fig. 6.38. Soldered bar with the correct amount of solder.

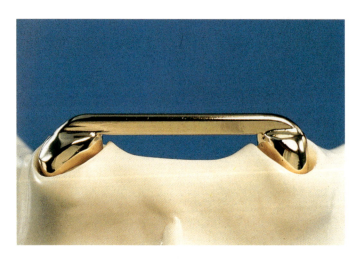

Fig. 6.39. The bar is rounded off at the ends and carefully polished.

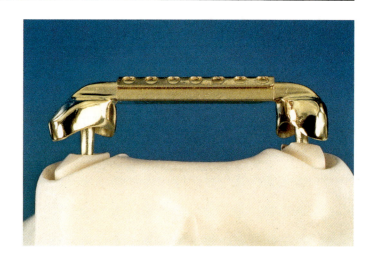

Fig. 6.40. Fit on the sleeve according to the space available.

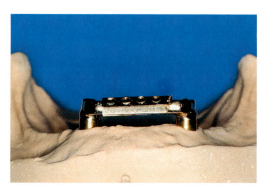

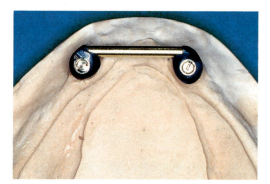

Fig. 6.41. An identical soldering procedure applies to implant copings.

Complications with bar retainers

While the operator has no choice over the position of abutment roots, this does not apply to implants. It is a common misconception that the construction of an overdenture does not require careful angulation and positioning of implants. Examples of misguided enthusiasm or implant placement before treatment planning are all too often found (Figs 6.42,

6.43) and correction at a late stage is almost impossible.

While correct design of the removable prosthesis minimises damage to the retaining clips, small clips are vulnerable, particularly when placed on distal cantilevers (Fig. 6.44). The easiest way to deal with this problem is to check for any excessive load that might be applied and then remove the clip with a minimum reduction of the surrounding acrylic

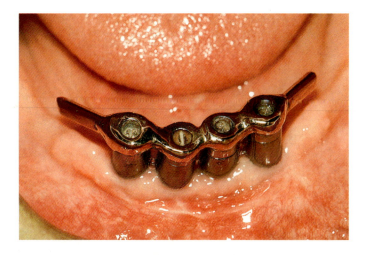

Fig. 6.42. An example of poor treatment planning that complicates plaque control and provides inadequate space for an anterior clip.

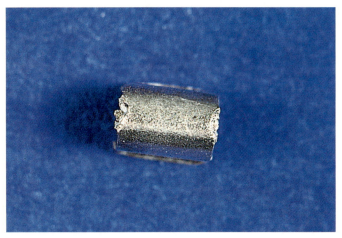

Fig. 6.43. Small clips are vulnerable to damage when placed on distal cantilevers.

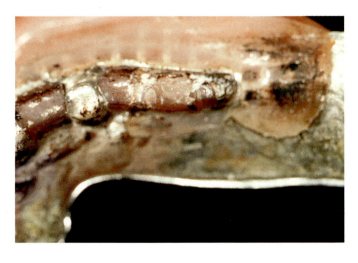

Fig. 6.44. Remove the clip with minimal reduction of the surrounding acrylic resin.

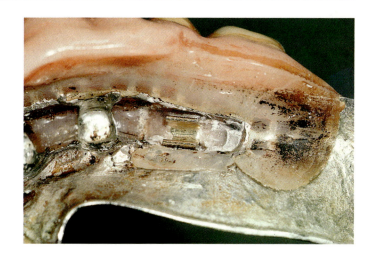

Fig. 6.45. The clip can now be simply replaced provided that its location is precise.

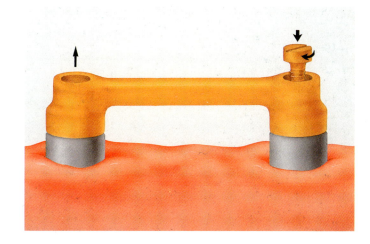

Fig. 6.46. Insert the screw at one end of the bar and check for any movement at the other as it is tightened; the screw is then removed and the procedure reversed.

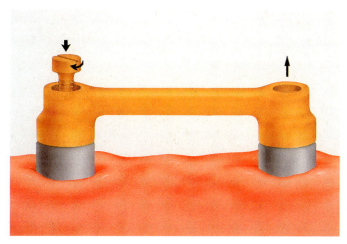

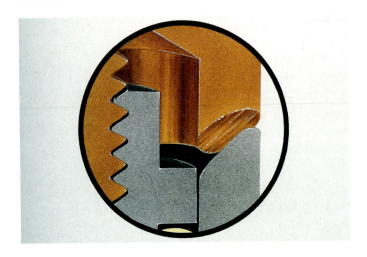

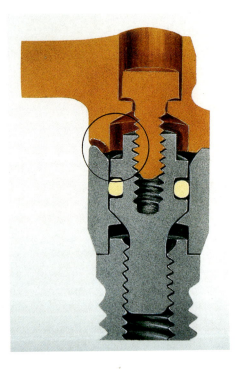

Fig. 6.47. Small mislocations either laterally or vertically can be difficult to detect.

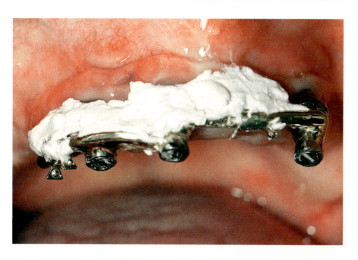

Fig. 6.48. Any mislocation will result in lack of passive fit. The bar must be cut and the sections located with resin or plaster. If an overall impression is to be employed, substitute guide pins for the gold screws. These guide pins should project through the impression tray in the normal manner.

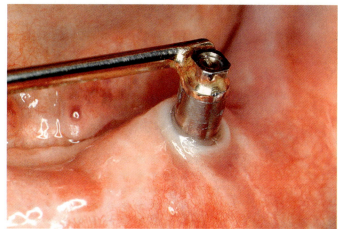

Fig. 6.49. Another example of poor treatment planning with the abutment penetrating mobile tissues. Note the lingual placement of the bar that was necessary and the poor solder joint.

resin (Fig. 6.45). A new clip can then be simply inserted into the depression left by the original and luted with a small amount of self-polymerising resin, carefully inserted around the tag (Fig. 6.46).

Experiments with strain gauges have shown that a surprising amount of strain can be induced within the bar assembly in the screw tightening process (Fig. 6.47). It is therefore extremely important to take every precaution to ensure that the superstructure fits the abutment (Fig. 6.48). To this end, it is normally wise practice to tighten the screw at one end first and see if there is any sign of lifting at the other. The screw can then be removed and the process repeated the other way round. If any rock or misfit is found, the bar must be sectioned and the pieces relocated and soldered (Fig. 6.49).

Where vertical space is limited, a

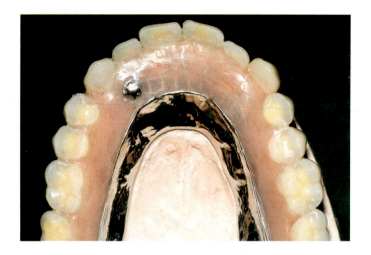

Fig. 6.50. Where vertical space is restricted, a section of the major connector can be used as an occlusal stop.

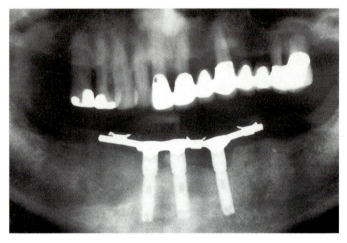

Fig. 6.51. Extensive cantilevered extensions, particularly on three abutments, are a prescription for failure. This failure is likely to happen sooner when there are supra-erupted natural teeth as antagonists.

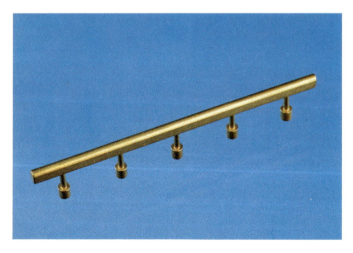

Fig. 6.52. The dummy Dolder bar that is incorporated within the master cast when duplicate or replacement dentures are to be made.

section of the major connector can be used both as an occlusal stop on one surface and as an occluding surface on the other (Fig 6.50). Needless to say, this is not a procedure that can be carried out at the last moment and highlights, once again, the importance of treatment planning. As for long cantilevered distal extensions the dangers of this approach have already been pointed out (Fig. 6.51).

Remaking a bar joint denture

With root supported overdentures, the main problem is reproducing the bar now firmly in the patient's mouth. With regard to the Dolder bars, and similar structures that run in a straight line, the procedure is as follows. A primary impression is made in a stock tray, this impression being made over the bar. The distance between the abutments should be measured and a length of bar and sleeve some 4 mm longer is obtained.

A closely adapted acrylic resin tray is then made on the cast of the primary impression and a slit cut in the tray overlying the bar. This slit should be wider than the sleeve that is to be fitted over the bar.

This new sleeve should next be placed in the patient's mouth, in conjunction with the appropriate spacer. Gaps between the base of the bar and the mucosa are blocked out with soft wax, or impression plaster, with the material extending

onto the free edge of the sleeve. The tray can now be checked for adaptation and border moulded. This tray must not impinge upon the bar/sleeve assembly. Zinc oxide–eugenol impression paste is then loaded into the tray, and the tray inserted in the mouth. When the material has set, excess paste that has flowed through the slit is removed while the tray is still in position. The sleeve is thus exposed and the slit filled with self-polymerising acrylic resin that unites the sleeve to the tray. When the tray has been removed, the sleeve will be locked in the impression. The spacer is now placed in the sleeve, followed by the bar analogue or a section of spare bar longer than the inter-abutment space. When the impression has been cast, the bar will be held in the artificial stone and the denture constructed upon it. Under no circumstances should the impression be cast without the bar in place, as the artificial stone will flow into the sleeve and result in the cast breaking when the impression is removed.

An alternative approach, and one to be preferred, is to employ a specially produced dummy bar that is incorporated in the master cast. Naturally, this is a technique that can only be employed where the original bar has not been bent and, like the Dolder bar, the manufacturer produces this special device (Fig. 6.52). After the impression has been made over the existing bar, taking the normal precautions to block out spaces under-

135

neath it, a section of dummy bar is selected and cut to a suitable length. This dummy bar is now carefully inserted into the corresponding section of the impression. The impression is now cast and the tagging that forms part of the dummy bar ensures that it is locked securely within the master cast. Laboratory produced bars, single sleeve bars that have been bent, and multiple sleeve bars are more difficult to reproduce, as a spare bar cannot be placed in the impression. A primary impression is made in an alginate material and a closely adapted acrylic resin tray produced on the cast of the impression. An elastomeric material, such as a polyether, can be used for the purpose, but spaces under the bar should be obliterated beforehand. The cast of this impression will now show the position of the bar, although the reproduction will not be exact. The sleeves, with corresponding spacers, are placed on the cast prior to duplication. These sleeves are placed to ensure an adequate thickness of acrylic resin around them when the denture framework is cast. At this point they are only being used as spacers for the denture framework.

The trial insertion can now be arranged in the conventional manner and once this has been established, the denture is processed. There are no sleeves in the denture base, only spaces for them. The location of the sleeves to the denture is carried out in the mouth, a difficult and exacting procedure. The spacers and corresponding sleeves, if applicable, are placed in the mouth and the denture positioned over them. It is essential that the denture seats correctly without binding upon any of the sleeves.

The next vital step is to ensure that all possible spaces under the bar are adequately obliterated. Impression plaster is excellent for this purpose, as it also ensures that the sleeve will not move during the location procedure. By carrying the plaster onto the tree end of the sleeve, one ensures that it will be free of acrylic resin. Small holes can now be drilled through the lingual aspects over the sleeves, so that excess resin flows through onto the lingual aspect of the denture rather than onto the impression surface. Any deficiencies in the acrylic resin around the sleeve can then be filled in with the denture out of the mouth. Once the location of the sleeves has been established, excess acrylic resin can be removed from the free end of the sleeves with a hot instrument. Burs should never be used for this purpose. The occlusion must then be checked and a check record procedure carried out.

Implant supported overdentures can be remade in the same manner, but an alternative approach is possible that takes advantage of the fact that the bar is screwed onto the implant abutment and not soldered to it. The initial clinical steps are identical to those set out before with the denture being completed, but with space to accommodate the sleeves. This prosthesis is then inserted and the borders and articulation checked. Locating the sleeves in the denture may be accomplished as follows. Small holes are drilled through the denture over each retaining screw. The screws are removed and guide pins of 10 mm substituted. Polyether adhesive is painted on the impression surface of the denture in the bar region and a polyether impression of this section is made by syringing the material under the bar, placing a small amount within the corresponding depression of the denture, and seating the prosthesis firmly in place. Once the impression has set, the guide pins are undone and the denture, with the bar firmly attached and correctly located, removed. Root analogues are attached to the gold cylinders, undercuts within the denture carefully blocked out and the impression cast. The sleeves can now be correctly located within the denture base, the access holes for the guide pins filled in and the denture completed. For practitioners with laboratories close by, this is a procedure that can be undertaken while the patient waits.

7   Impression procedures

Introduction

Surveys of overdenture results highlight the importance of an accurate working impression. The difficulty of the procedure is often underestimated, particularly in the case of implant supported prostheses which are sometimes, but mistakenly, thought to be simpler to construct than the corresponding fixed prosthesis. If one is to construct an implant supported fixed prosthesis, the details of the surrounding soft tissues are of interest but they are certainly not load bearing. With an implant supported overdenture, these details are extremely important to prevent unnecessary and excessive leverages on the implant.

Impressions for overdentures on roots or for implants have three distinct requirements:

1. An impression of the entire denture bearing area.
2. An impression of the root preparations. For implant procedures, an impression coping representing the head of the implant or of the implant abutment will be employed (Fig 7.1).
3. A correct relationship between 1 and 2.

Any inadequacy in the above must produce serious consequences.

The distortions that can occur are sometimes referred to as total, when the entire impression is affected, or relative in which sections are mal-related. Significant distortions of either type are unacceptable. In relating implant components to one another, inaccuracies of less than 30 microns are normally required. This applies to distortions both in the vertical plane and lateral areas.

It is apparent that the health of the oral tissues must be sound before impression procedures are undertaken. This may involve adapting and correcting previously unsatisfactory dentures, together with using tissue conditioning procedures. With all root supported overdentures, the importance of sound periodontal tissues is vital to the success of the restoration. An adequate zone of attached gingivae and reasonable sulcus depth are other important requisites for a good prognosis.

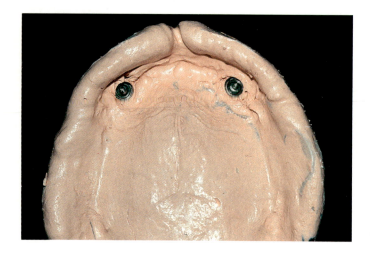

Fig. 7.1. Impressions for overdentures on roots or implants involve three distinct stages. An impression of the entire denture bearing area is required, together with an impression of the root preparations or implants. Finally, these two components must be correctly related to one another.

Impressions of the denture bearing area

Most complete overdentures are supported by roots or implants, but a large measure of support is derived from the mucosa. Base extension principles are similar to those of complete dentures. Exceptions are rare, but include situations where multiple implants have been placed in a jaw or where four or more teeth remain and comparatively rigid telescopic retainers are employed. Where mucogingival surgery has been undertaken, sufficient time must be allowed for healing before impression procedures are carried out. An average period of 6 weeks should be allowed to elapse. For implants, about 2 weeks after abutment connection should suffice.

An adequately extended final impression is a prerequisite for any satisfactory prosthesis. For the denture to be stable, occlusal loads must be distributed as widely as possible and the forces of both adhesion and cohesion developed to their maximum. To resist vertical loads, coverage of the buccal shelf area of the mandible is essential, whilst palatal coverage of the maxillae plays a similar role. If the impression features some mocosal displacement, the impression surface of the denture will be contoured to the shape that the mucosa will assume under load. While slight displacement of the denture bearing mucosa is a necessary part of the impression procedure, no displacement of the gingival margins should take place. The denture base will therefore need to make a scarcely perceptible movement before occlusal load and mucosal resistance reach equilibrium. Movement of the denture base around the roots or implants will then be reduced to a minimum. Such an impression technique will also help in the development of a border seal, necessary for the production of adequate retention.

Denture base extension

Correct extension of the complete lower denture base is not only essential if the retentive forces are to be developed to the best advantage, but also necessary for maximum stability. However, it is support from the buccal shelf area that is so important if the underlying implants or roots are to be shielded from excessive torques. The directions in which denture flanges run are usually determined by the contours of the underlying bone, and by the extension of the soft tissues. In the posterior lingual region this does not hold true, since it is necessary to allow the mylohyoid muscle freedom of movement. In this area, the inclination of the lingual flange may be incorrect. For example, one often sees poorly extended complete lower dentures that appear to balance precariously on the edentulous ridge. Commonly, the lingual flanges rest on the mylohyoid ridges, where they cause trauma and subject the denture to a displacing force whenever the patient moves the tongue. The problem is not one of simple extension, as the base is already over-extended in this region; nor will reduction of the flange help matters. The answer lies in a lingually inclin-ed, fully extended, flange with a border seal, allowing the mylohyoid muscle freedom of movement underneath.

The mylohyoid muscle probably causes more difficulty in denture construction than any other single muscle. The posterior part of the mylohyoid muscle guards the entrance to the retromylohyoid fossa and it is this part that so frequently causes difficulty. The mylohyoid muscle forms the floor of the mouth. Anteriorly, it is attached fairly low to the internal aspect of the mandible. However, in the premolar region the level of attachment rises sharply, and it is from this point to its posterior border that the mylohyoid is related to the denture base. When the mylohyoid is relaxed, its more posterior fibres run almost vertically downwards to the hyoid bone; when it contracts, the hyoid bone is raised and the direction of the fibres become more horizontal.

A vertical denture flange adapted to the mylohyoid muscle at rest will be displaced as soon as the mylohyoid muscle contracts. This occurs however short the flange. The resulting trauma may be quite substantial, for if attachments are being used, these hold the denture firmly in place, and the occlusion of the teeth will press the denture back on to the contracted mylohyoid muscle. It is therefore necessary to incline the denture flange lingually around the contracted mylohyoid muscle so that this muscle can contract under the flange. Once the flange is behind the posterior border of the mylohyoid muscles, it may be turned back into the retromylohyoid fossa. It is true that a flange adapted to a contracted mylohyoid muscle may leave a potential space when this muscle is at rest, but as the seal is maintained in the reflection of the lingual mucosa, this potential space is unlikely to be of clinical significance.

When the mouth is opened wide the appearance of a flat edentulous ridge can be misleading. The base of the tongue, in contact with the retromylohyoid fossa and lateral aspect of the retromolar pad, usually obliterates the lingual vestibule, but careful examination of this area using a mouth mirror, while the tongue is moved, provides a better evaluation of the space available.

It is normal practice to consider the placement of the border but not the denture border thickness. A useful diagnostic aid is the estimation of the high and low levels of the floor of the mouth. The patient who has the least movement has the best prognosis, because it is easier to establish and maintain a good border seal. Patients with square jaws and short thick necks will often have hyoid bones that move very little during speech and swallowing: patients with tapering jaws and longer necks often have hyoid bones that demonstrate far more movement. An excellent diagnostic aid is to feel the floor of the mouth in function. The index finger should touch the floor of the mouth around the first molar region, with the maxillary denture in place. The patient is asked to swallow. The finger can be placed anteriorly and then posteriorly so that the various regions can be evaluated for potential border length, width, and sublingual extensions.

In the maxillae the primary support areas lie on the hard palate either side of the midline (Fig. 7.2). It is important to record details of the entire palate even if the operator may feel that sufficient root or implant support exists to allow a subsequent reduction of denture base coverage. A complete palatal impression will facilitate the precise delineation of the posterior denture border Furthermore, wherever the posterior border is placed, full palatal coverage for jaw relation records and even trial insertions will simplify manipulation of the trial bases.

The tuberosity region is another problem area, as recording details of both tuberosities together with their sulci is essential. Even multiple implant supported overdentures with reduced palatal coverage should cover the tuberosities. The failure rate of maxillary implants is significantly higher than those placed in the mandible, and for this reason every effort should be made to reduce torques applied. The primary support areas of the mandible lie on the buccal shelf (Fig. 7.3).

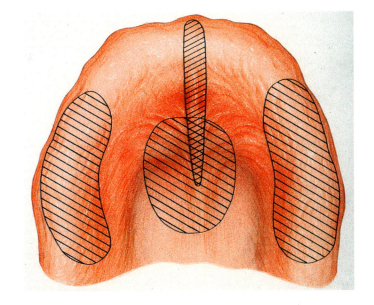

Fig. 7.2. In the upper jaw the primary support areas lie on the hard palate either side of the midline. Reduced denture base coverage in these regions requires adequate support from other structures – usually implants.

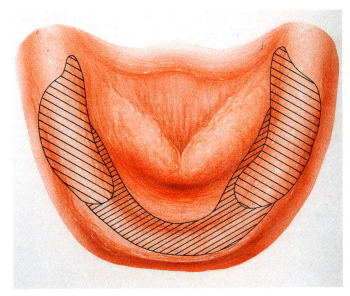

Fig. 7.3. The primary support areas of the mandible lie on the buccal shelves.

Selecting the tray

Since one starts a primary impression procedure with a stock tray and hopes to finish with a well adapted impression, it is hardly necessary to point out the importance of a good selection of correctly contoured metal trays. So often overlooked is the influence of the tray upon the contours of the impression (Fig. 7.4). The distance an impression material can flow beyond the tray is limited, while the direction in which it flows is influenced by the tray as well as by the mucosa.

One of the common faults of a lower stock tray is a short, straight lingual flange which directs the impression material vertically downwards and does not guide it posteriorly into the retromylohyoid fossa. Quite frequently, this results in displacement of the mylohyoid muscle and distortion of the border structure.

Another common mistake is to employ a stock tray that distorts the sulcus, particularly the labial sulcus. The impression of the sulcus is bulky, but inadequately extended. The tray constructed to the cast will reproduce this error and the impression made in it can only follow these contours. As a result, the denture will have a thick labial flange. Although this flange can be reduced, the extension will be inadequate and the border seal compromised (Fig. 7.5). A simple technique has been well described by Neill and Nairn (1990). The initial compound impression is made with the mylohyoid muscles contracted, and the patient's tongue firmly pressed forward against the anterior section of the palate. The impression is then removed, chilled, and the bulk reduced with a sharp knife. At least 2 mm of compound is removed from the surface overlying the mylohyoid muscles and from the surface over the buccal aspects of the roots. Compound is notoriously prone to displace soft tissues and fraenae, so that extra bulk must be carefully removed. The extension is then checked in the mouth and, when satisfactory, the surface is painted with adhesive and an alginate wash impression made. The cast from this impression provides details of the denture-bearing area and shows the position of the root preparations (Fig. 7.6).

A closely adapted acrylic resin tray can be made on this cast. If transfer copings are to be employed, holes are cut over the roots slightly larger than the roots and their gingival margins. The lingual flange should be about 4 mm thick in the molar region so there is room available to relieve the impression surface from the mylohyoid muscles (Fig. 7.7). Posteriorly, the lingual flange may be thinned slightly and turned laterally into the retromylohyoid space. The tray must be completely rigid, to eliminate any distortion when the impression is made. Three stub handles are useful; the anterior one for positioning the tray in the mouth, the posterior ones for holding the tray

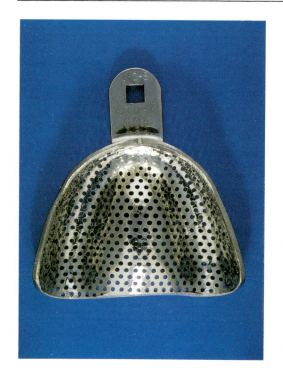
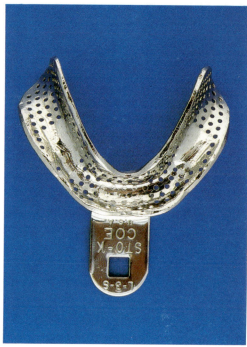

Fig. 7.4. Well contoured stock strays are an important prerequisite to impression procedures.

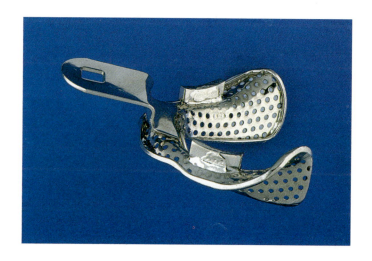

Fig. 7.5. The STO-K system is an example.

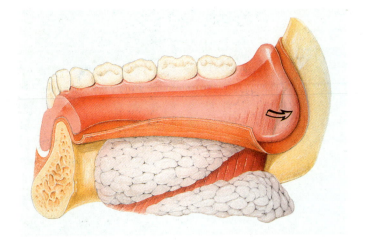

Fig. 7.6. Simplified diagram to show the relationship of the mylohyoid muscle to the denture base.

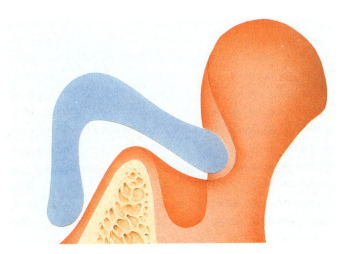

Fig. 7.7. A common distortion of the labial sulcus. This will lead to the construction of a poorly extended and bulky denture base. The thickness can be reduced, but it will not be adapted to the sulcus.

in place when the impression is made.

The rear stub handles should be placed slightly buccal to the midline of the ridge, so that the impression load is taken by the buccal shelf area – one of the primary stress bearing regions of the edentulous mouth. The anterior stub handle is employed for positioning the tray in the mouth.

Finger holds are placed in the handles, as the tray can become slippery. Ideally, the labial surface of the handle and tray should resemble the contour of the completed denture, so that the labial sulcus is faithfully reproduced and not, as one often sees, with a large handle that displaces the lower lip and distorts the labial sulcus (Figs. 7.8–7.10).

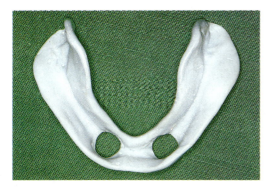

Fig. 7.8. A closely adapted acrylic resin tray should be made on the cast of the primary impression. If transfer copings are to be employed, holes should be cut over the roots to leave both these roots and the surrounding area uncovered. A window may be substituted for individual holes where necessary.

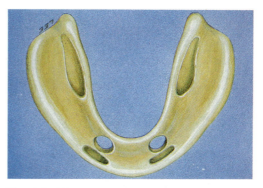

Fig. 7.9. Where root supported overdentures are concerned, the tray should be relieved from the area covering the mylohyoid muscles and from the buccal aspects of the roots.

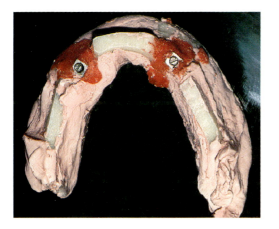

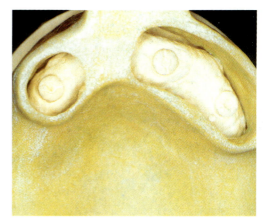

Fig. 7.10. Anterior stub handles should not distort the labial sulcus. They cannot usually be employed when more than two anterior implants have been placed. The posterior handles should be placed in positions corresponding with the artificial molar teeth.

All the surfaces of the impression tray should duplicate those of the completed denture. It is not just the extension of the border that matters, it is the thickness of the border and the contour of the buccal and lingual surfaces. Although the basic extension of the impression tray may be correct, border moulding techniques should be employed to perfect the seal.

Impressions of the edentulous maxilla are rather more straightforward. As with the mandible, it is important to record details of the entire denture bearing area. Common trouble spots include the tuberosities, where a poorly adapted tray will not provide adequate extension. Conversely, a border that is too thick in this region will be displaced by the coronoid process of the mandible during lateral jaw movements.

While all operators would agree upon the significance of the labial sulcus, many fail to appreciate the problems that may arise from the majority of stock trays. The facial aspects of many premaxillae are concave, whereas most stock trays have a vertical labial flange. The unwary operator will see a rolled border in the impression and be lulled into a false sense of security.

In fact, what has been recorded is a distorted reproduction of the labial sulcus. The flange of the tray will have displaced the lip facially on widening the sulcus by a significant extent but also shortening it. If this error is not corrected at the working impression stage, it will result in a short fat labial flange, unsatisfactory for a complete denture, but particularly unfortunate for an overdenture where labial contours are so critical. Reduction of the flange thickness at this late stage may reduce the labial distortion, but will result in lack of border seal. If the labial flange has been inadvertently distorted by the primary impression, the custom tray will need to be correctly contoured and then border moulded where it is short. Under normal circumstances the posterior border of the denture will be the vibrating line.

The tray will require to be accurately contoured to provide details of the entire tuberosity regions and sulci. There remains the question of the relatively hard midline area of the palate which may require some relief.

Impressions of roots and implants

Although considered separately, these impressions normally form part of the overall locating impression to relate these structures to the denture bearing areas. In order to prevent undue repetition, the actual techniques are described together with the locating procedures themselves.

Locating procedures

The impression of the denture bearing area is, naturally, critical to the success of the overdenture. However, unlike the complete denture the overdenture gains support from underlying roots or implants. This produces an additional complication, as the impression of the edentulous area must be related to the impressions of the roots or implants together with any restoration that may be placed on them. For descriptive purposes, the various locating procedures commonly employed have been divided into two groups and their relative merits considered.

Locating procedures before denture construction

(a) "All-in-one" impression (Figs. 7.11, 7.12).
(b) Completing the metalwork of the root preparations and luting them in place before making an overall impression (Fig. 7.13).
(c) Completing metalwork for abutment preparations and placing them without a luting agent. These restorations are removed or subsequently placed in an overall locating impression.
(d) Transfer coping techniques. These are particularly relevant for osseointegration procedures.

Locating procedures following denture construction

(a) Laboratory processing.
(b) Intra-oral processing.

The main applications of this approach rest with the use of attachment retained overdentures.

Locating procedures before denture construction

"All-in-one" impression

Tempting as it may be, an impression of root preparations and of the entire edentulous area is remarkably difficult to obtain. The relatively long setting time of elastomeric materials, to say nothing of their expense, appears to deter operators from multiple attempts. However, even a successful impression can be rendered quite useless for denture construction when the cast is sectioned to produce individual dies.

Completing metalwork of the root preparations and luting them before an overall impression of the edentulous area is made

This approach is particularly useful when individual precious metal root copings or other castings are to be constructed. Two impressions are required, one of the abutment preparations and a subsequent impression of the completed abutment preparations for the overdenture. It is important to ensure that the initial

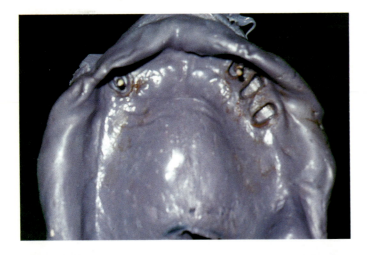

Fig. 7.11. An all-in-one impression is difficult to obtain. Subsequent die production is likely to render the cast useless for denture construction unless great care is taken.

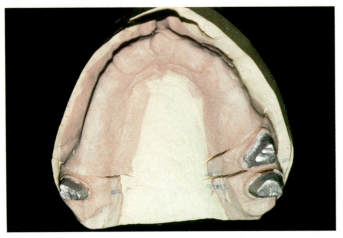

Fig. 7.12. Master cast showing damage that precludes its use for denture construction.

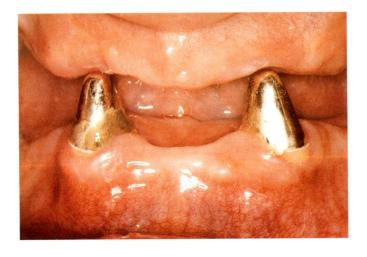

Fig. 7.13. Where simple gold copings are involved, they can be luted first before making an overal impression. The operator must ensure that adequate vertical space exists or this type of mishap could easily occur.

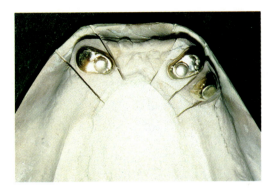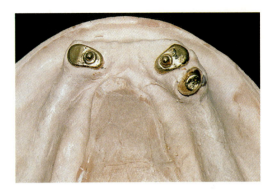

Fig. 7.14. The double impression system is versatile. It is particularly useful for attachment retained root supported overdentures. The first impression is made of the root preparations but must include the entire edentulous area to allow the path of insertion of the denture to be determined. The root restorations are placed unluted in the mouth and removed in the second stage impression. The cast of this impression is used for the construction of the overdenture.

impression of the abutment preparations must cover the entire edentulous area, so as to allow the path of the overdenture to be determined and the wax-up of the copings completed in alignment with this path (Fig. 7.14).

Completing metalwork of abutment preparations and placing them unluted before an overall impression of the edentulous area is made

This valuable and popular technique works well with most stud and bar retainers and even root copings. The metalwork is made on an initial impression that covers the entire denture bearing area and this allows the path of insertion of the overdenture to be planned. The cast of this impression is sectioned to allow individual dies to be prepared. There

are, however, important modifications that may be necessary. Aligning and soldering attachments to the root restorations before the artificial tooth position has been decided is not normally recommended, particularly when bar attachments are considered or in Class II, Division 2 malocclusions. Normally, the root restoration only would be completed, leaving part of the sprue projecting to allow it to be removed in the impression. In these situations the attachments would be aligned and soldered after the trial insertion. Actually completing the metalwork at this early stage implies confidence that adequate vertical and bucco-lingual space will exist when the tooth position is selected.

Once the copings or attachments have been completed, another custom tray is constructed, spaced over

151

the metalwork, but close fitting else-where. An overall impression is made in this tray and the unluted metal castings picked up in the impression material. Where simple dome shaped copings are employed, it is advisable to leave a small amount of the sprue attached in order to assist in locating the metalwork in the impression. These metal castings are incorporated in the master cast on which the denture is subsequently constructed. The metal castings are not removed from this cast until the denture has been completed, so that location between castings and denture base is assured.

One word of warning. It is important to assess the amount of vertical and buccolingual space available before using attachments or any space occupying retainer. Failure to carry out this important step may result in the metal showing through the occlusal surface of the denture, thereby spoiling the appearance and rendering it liable to fracture. Time spent in constructing the impression that forms the foundation of the restoration can only be considered a sound investment.

Transfer coping techniques

Although a dated method now, the principles of these techniques are important and for this reason they are described at some length. Transfer copings are used extensively where osseointegrated fixtures are concerned. As for root supported over-dentures, it allows the operator to concentrate on each individual root preparation at a time until satisfied with the impression obtained. Impression compound or an elastomeric material placed in a copper band is usually employed for the impression, with a stainless steel or resin dowel to provide an accurate impression of the root canal preparation. Impressions can be repeated fairly quickly until the operator is content.

A copper plated die is produced, although Velmix (Vel-Mix Stone Sybron, Kerr UK Ltd, Peterborough) is an acceptable alternative, and on this die the transfer coping is constructed. Metal transfer copings will not distort and give consistent results, but they are time consuming to make and expensive. Nowadays, one generally employs a hard resin transfer coping made of a substance such as Duralay (Duralay Inlay Pattern Resin, Reliance Dental Mfg, Worth, Ill.), but this must be used with great care to ensure correct seating without application of excessive loads.

Preformed stainless steel dowels should be used if they form part of the dowel kit and the operator must ensure that the resin engages the anti-rotation slot so that not the slightest movement may be made in the mouth. The shape of the projection should be slightly undercut. Transfer copings are placed on each of the preparations and when the operator is satisfied that they seat with accuracy, they can be set aside while he concentrates on obtaining a satisfactory impression of the edentulous area. A closely adapted custom made tray will have been produced on the primary impression and this tray can now be inserted using Kelly's Paste (Kelly's Impression Paste, Type II Soft, Teledyne Getz, Elk Grove Village, Ill. 60007, USA), or another suitable zinc oxide–eugenol material. The first attempt should be considered a diagnostic impression to correct minor inaccuracies of the tray. It is unlikely that the first impression would be satisfactory, and the impression is repeated, with modification of the tray, until the operator feels that the next impression is likely to be of an adequate standard. The transfer copings are now placed over their respective roots, the impression tray loaded with impression paste, and inserted over the transfer copings which project through the holes in the tray. The impression material itself is too weak to connect copings and tray, and once the material has hardened, a layer of self-polymerising resin can be placed over the impression material, linking the coping directly with the tray. By carrying out the procedure in this manner, the self-polymerising resin is kept away from the gingivae, but it should be remembered that the eugenol in the impression material is likely to retard the polymerisation of the resin so that extra time should be allowed for the process to take place. Impression plaster placed between coping and

tray is a suitable alternative and has a faster setting time.

Once the copings are united with the impression tray, the entire assembly can be removed from the mouth. The dies are then carefully located on their respective copings and the impression poured. The cast obtained from this impression, the master cast, is an accurate reproduction of the denture bearing mucosa, the gingival margins, the root preparations and the relations between these structures. On this master cast the occlusal rims are made and the denture finally processed.

The versatility provided by this approach helps offset the additional time that may be involved in the construction of transfer copings and the fact that at least two appointments will be required to obtain the master impression. This method can be used when stud or bar attachments are to be employed. It enables both the metalwork and the final denture to be constructed on the same master cast so that the location of the two sections of the attachments is established in the laboratory on one cast. The margin for error is small.

At the next clinical visit, the operator can check the retention of the dowel-retained restorations, leave these unluted, and place the denture over them to ensure the location is correct. As a rule of thumb, these unluted restorations should stay in place when the denture is removed, thereby demonstrating that the chances of accidental displacement when these restorations have been luted are minimal. Particular attention has to be paid to the preparation of the dies that are placed in their respective transfer copings and the technician must be able to remove these dies without damage to the surrounding master cast. If inadequate attention is paid to this important detail, the master cast will be deficient in the critical area that surrounds the root preparations and this will be reflected in a poorly adapted overdenture.

Osseointegration procedures

For most patients the operator will be making an impression over the transmucosal abutments. The first and essential step is to ensure that these abutments are correctly located on their respective implants, and radiographic confirmation is essential (Figs. 7.15, 7.16).

Most implant techniques are based on employing the manufacturer's transfer coping, which is placed over the transmucosal abutment and secured with a screw. Accuracy can then be assured provided that there is no intervening debris. In rare situations such as unusual implant angulation, it may be necessary to record the location of the actual head of the implant itself using a specially produced transfer coping for this purpose. This will be discussed later (Figs. 7.17–7.19).

A primary impression using alginate in a stock tray is made. A complication here is the adaptation of the stock tray, as the healing abutments will prevent complete seating of the stock tray. If the discrepancy is small, the problem may be overcome using soft wax to border mould the tray, accepting the minor distortion of the sulci that must inevitably occur. Where the projection above the mucosa is larger, the operator will be obliged to use a tray designed for the dentate mouth. In these circumstances distortion of the sulci must occur, and the tray produced on the cast will require extensive border moulding.

In constructing the laboratory-produced tray, the operator has to provide a window sufficiently large to accommodate the transmucosal abutment and the transfer coping. Additional spacing should be provided, as the transfer copings may be located to one another with a material such as Duralay which may interfere with seating the impression tray unless provision has been made for it. Where implants have been closely opposed, one window is normally made and the location between the transfer copings assured with Duralay applied in small increments. Where widely spaced implants have been located, the tray is made with two holes through which the transfer copings project (Fig. 7.20). The location between the two copings is assured after the overall impression has been made. Fast

Fig. 7.15. Radiographic confirmation of the abutment implant interface is essential. In this instance the abutment screw felt tight but the mislocation is clearly visible.

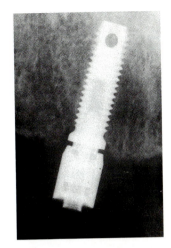
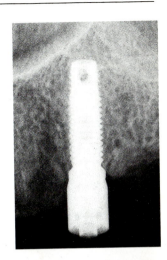

Fig. 7.16. Correction of the mislocation.

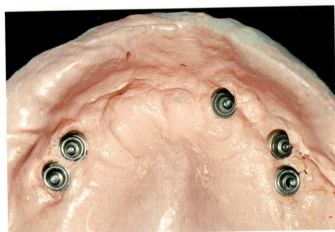

Fig. 7.17. The transfer coping technique is normally employed for implant supported overdentures.

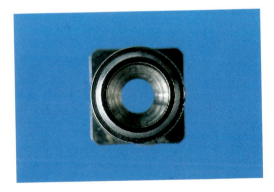
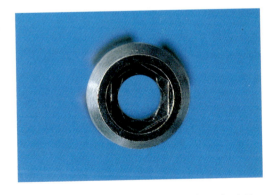

Fig. 7.18. Transfer coping for transmucosal abutments. Note the circular internal profile.

Fig. 7.19. Transfer coping for head of the implant. Note the receptacle to engage the hexagonal projection on the implant.

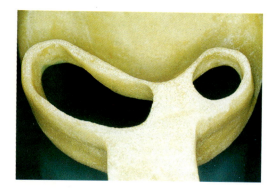
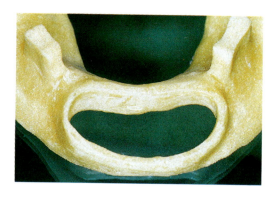
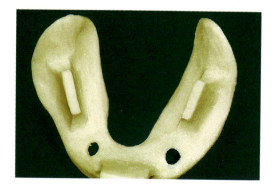

Fig. 7.20. The shape of the window is dictated by the implant positions. Where the span between the implants does not permit direct connection of the copings, the copings are united to the tray. Duralay can be employed for this purpose. Fast setting impression plaster is a quicker method of locking the coping to the impression tray.

setting impression plaster is normally the most convenient, although Duralay can be employed, bearing in mind that the setting time is likely to be greatly increased if placed over a zinc oxide–eugenol type impression paste. Either way, the dental surgery assistant will need to apply additional material over the copings to ensure that they are firmly united. The relationship of the copings to one another is critical and leaves no room for error. In practice, the actual location of the copings is undertaken once the accuracy of the acrylic resin tray has been assured.

Since the impression procedure is relatively time consuming, the use of this diagnostic impression in the custom tray before the placement of transfer copings is strongly recommended. On the basis of the diagnostic impression, the operator can make adjustments to the tray and be assured that when the definitive impression is actually made, there is a very good chance that it will be acceptable. The diagnostic impression should be made, the tray adapted, and then cleaned before the transfer copings are placed in the mouth. Since titanium is relatively soft and easily damaged or burnished by opposing teeth or even a denture, healing caps should always be placed over the transmucosal abutments and only removed for the impression procedure (Figs. 7.21, 7.22).

Two contours of impression copings are available, squared and tapered. The squared type of coping is designed to be removed in the impression tray and it is this method that is normally preferred for all overdenture construction. The tapered coping remains in place while the impression is removed and is then repositioned in the impression outside the mouth. The square shaped coping removed in the impression is usually the more accurate of the two methods.

At least three lengths of screw are available to secure impression copings onto the transmucosal abutment. In the case of the Branemark (Branemark components, Nobelpharma) system the screws, sometimes called guiding pins, are 10 mm, 15 mm, and 20 mm long, the shortest being virtually flush with the top of the coping (Fig. 7.23). The longer the screw, the further it will project through the impression tray and the easier it is to loosen after the impression material has been set. The drawback is that the impression tray has to be manipulated over the screw before it can be seated in place, and so the screw length is selected according to the amount of space available. The shortest screws may well be required in the case of maxillary overdentures opposing natural teeth, and in these instances, one should take every precaution to ensure that the heads of the screws are easily found and not buried under a mass of impression material, as it is impossibe to remove the impression tray until all the screws have been completely loosened (Fig. 7.24). Attempting to remove the impression tray with one screw only partly loosened can be painful and cause damage. Always ensure that the screw is undone. This can be achieved by pulling on the screw head with tweezers to make certain that movement is possible. If the head of the screw is surrounded by impression material or access is difficult, continuing to unscrew the pin until a pronounced click is felt, and repeated, should ensure that coping and abutment are truly separated.

Once the impression has been removed from the mouth, an analogue representing the transmucosal abutment is carefully placed over the transfer coping. If impression plaster has been used for locating purposes, this may require the analogue to be placed, removed and any loose plaster blown away before it is finally seated on to the impression coping and the screw tightened (Fig. 7.25). If Duralay is employed as the locating medium, additional curing time will be required due to the effect of the Eugenol in the impression material (Fig. 7.26). When a polyether or

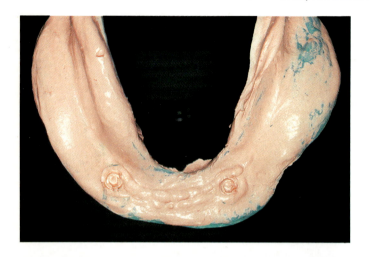

Fig. 7.21. Before securing the impression copings, the tray is corrected with a series of diagnostic impressions.

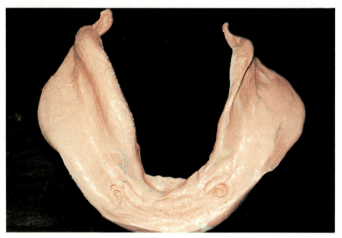

Fig. 7.22. Following the initial correction, the rolled border in the right mylohyoid region is deficient.

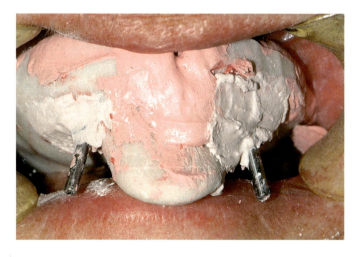

Fig. 7.23. Longer guide pins are easier to unscrew than shorter ones, but there has to be sufficient space to manipulate the tray over the guidepins. Impression plaster is a rapid and convenient method of connecting copings and trays.

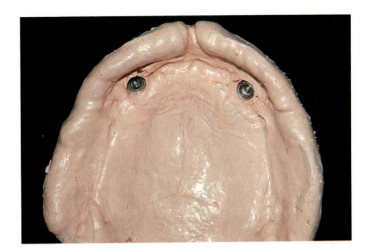

Fig. 7.24. After removal, check to ensure that copings and tray are united.

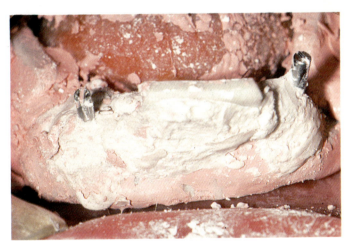

Fig. 7.25. A similar approach used for mandibular impressions.

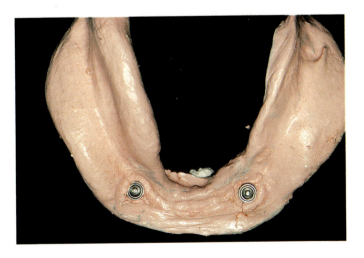

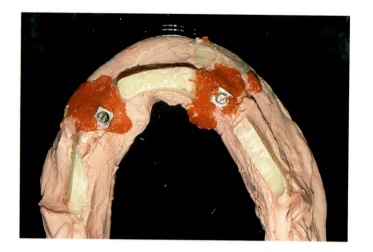

Fig. 7.26. Duralay can be employed to locate the copings to the impression tray.

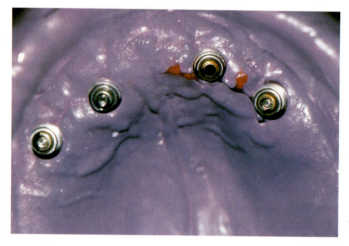

Fig. 7.27.(a) Polyether (Impregum) or silicone impression materials may be used and Duralay employed to locate the copings.

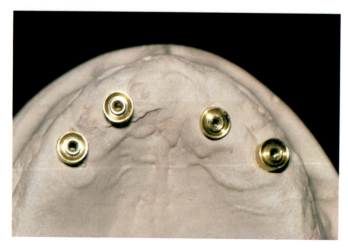

Fig. 7.27.(b) Master Cast.

silicone impression is employed, this does not apply (Fig. 7.27). Each of the root analogues is carefully positioned in this manner before the impression is cast. It is normally wise practice for the operator to carry out this procedure in case one of the transfer copings is not adequately secure within the impression. This will be discovered as the screw connecting the coping and analogue is tightened and the impression can be remade at the same appointment. Angled abutments are normally best avoided. They complicate plaque control and construction of the prosthesis and may possibly lead to stress concentrations. However, sometimes their use is inevitable.

Manufacturers normally recommend that the angled abutment TMA is placed in the mouth over the implant concerned. A radiograph is essential to make sure it is correctly seated. Angled abutments require special conical shaped healing caps and impression copings (Figs. 7.28). A conical shaped abutment analogue is also part of the system. For practical purposes, the impression procedures are identical to those with conventional abutments apart from the special components. Later on, when the metal work is constructed, a matching conical shaped precious metal cap is available. This method is very straightforward to use, the only drawback being that the operator has to decide, in the mouth, the exact angulation required, and select the correct height of abutment

where a choice is available. Since the abutment may be rotated and secured in one of 12 positions, and there may be more than one angled abutment involved, it is not always easy to make the correct decision at the chairside. If, for any reason, the restoration is subsequently dismantled, reassembling the abutments in their correct relationship can be remarkably difficult.

When faced with angled abutments, many experienced operators would prefer to position the abutments in the laboratory. The alignment can be assessed with the aid of a surveyor and the relationship of the abutment together with its superstructure checked against the position of the artificial teeth. These are very considerable advantages, well worth the additional clinical complexity (Figs. 7.29, 7.30).

Handling angled abutments can be made easier if a specially produced holder is screwed into the hole of the gold screw. An alternative is to use a guide pin. Both methods allow the operator to carry the abutment into place before the central screw is tightened. The first step requires an impression of the implant head, not the transmucosal abutment, and a specially produced transfer coping that fits over the head is required. With the Branemark system, this coping incorporates a hexagonal depression to fit over the corresponding projection of the implant. Graduations on the coping help assess the depth of the implant

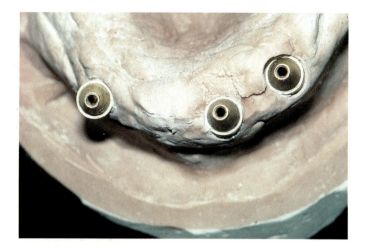

Fig. 7.28. Malaligned implants require angled abutments. The conventional approach is to place the angled abutment on the implant, and employ a specially made impression coping and abutment analogue to produce the master cast.

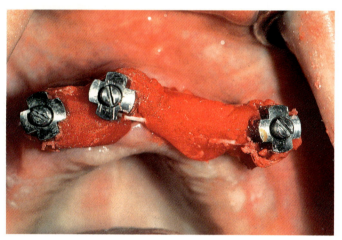

Fig. 7.29. If the abutments are to be aligned in the laboratory, and this is normally to be preferred, it is necessary to make an impression of the heads of the implants using single tooth impression copings. Duralay should be added in small increments.

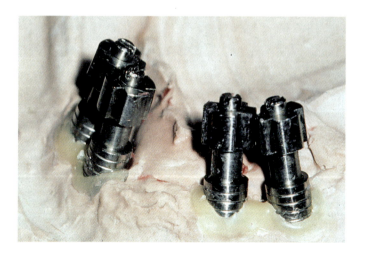

Fig. 7.30. Lingually inclined copings on the master cast demonstrate the tongue cramping that would occur with conventional abutments.

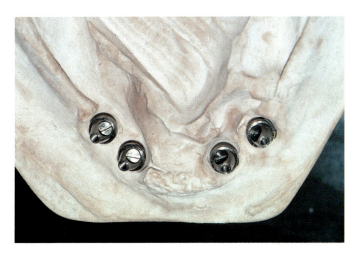

Fig. 7.31. Angled abutments have been placed on the master cast.

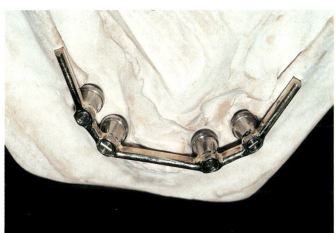

Fig. 7.32. The bar assembly showing the tongue space that has been produced.

beneath the mucosa, although this measurement can be obtained from the master cast. Since the adaptation of the transfer coping to the implant is critical and cannot be examined visually, a radiograph must be taken to ensure that it is correctly seated. The transfer coping is incorporated within the impression in the normal manner, but a specially manufactured implant analogue has to be employed, representing the head of the implant rather than the transmucosal abutment. A soft material is normally poured around the transfer coping before the impression is cast, but this is not absolutely essential (Figs. 7.31, 7.32).

When the impression has been cast, the operator then has in his possession a replica of the patient's jaw incorporating the head of the implant. Jaw relation records and trial insertion procedures are undertaken with

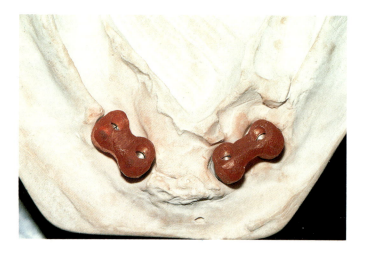

Fig. 7.33. Duralay copings have been made to locate the angled abutments in their correct relationships. Note the access for the screw.

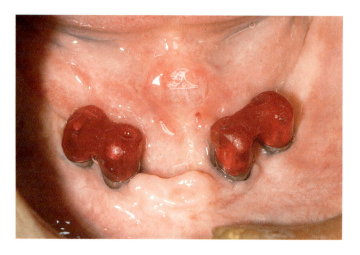

Fig. 7.34. Following sterilisation of abutments, these copings assist in the correct orientation of the abutments on their respective implants. They should be preserved in the patient's records in case it should prove necessary to dismantle the bar assembly.

this cast so that the ideal tooth position can be established. A silicone mask is prepared so that the position of the teeth is recorded and the abutments can then be placed on the implant analogues in the best possible relationship. Attempting to complete the superstructure before the trial insertion is a dangerous gamble when angled abutments are necessary. The drawback to this approach is that the operator has to place the angled abutments in the mouth in the same relationship that exists on the master cast. A positioning device made of Duralay is more than useful for this purpose and also facilitates any subsequent maintenance procedures. It will be necessary to sterilise the abutments before placement in the mouth and to take radiographs to ensure that they are correctly located on their respective implants (Figs. 7.33, 7.34).

Restricted vertical space

A similar approach can be employed where available vertical space may present a problem. Vertical space limitations are best assessed at the treatment planning stage, but the severity of the problem may not be appreciated. Previous complete dentures can provide a valuable clue and should be examined carefully. For example, the imprint of lower incisors on the thin palate of a complete denture is a danger sign to be taken seriously (Fig. 7.35). Despite the production of surgical stents showing the artificial tooth position required, bone contours may not allow ideal position or angulation of the implants. An impression technique providing the operator with the maximum versatility is therefore required. Once the transmucosal abutments have been placed on the implants, an important decision has already been made.

Rather than inserting the abutments and then making an impression over these components, more control over the end result can be obtained if an impression is made of the actual heads of the implants. This allows both the selection of the abutments and the planning of the superstructure to be carried out on the master cast with the aid of the trial insertion. Working in this manner and seeing the position of the artificial teeth and their relationship to the heads of the implants allows one to determine with precision the space available.

The first step is a diagnostic impression made with the healing abutments in place. This helps the operator make corrections to the tray (Fig. 7.36). When it is next employed in the more time-consuming master impression, a satisfactory result will be more likely at the first attempt. The diagnostic impression is used only to perfect the impression tray, and once the operator is satisfied with the tray contours the impression material is removed from it.

The healing abutments can now be removed (Fig. 7.37) and single tooth impression copings placed over each of the implants. Care must be taken to ensure that the hexagonal receptacle in the coping precisely engages the corresponding projection of the implant head and a radiograph is recommended (Fig. 7.38) to check the relationship. The impression copings should be rigidly and accurately located to each other (Fig. 7.39). Impression plaster is a convenient material. Duralay may be used for small spans if used incrementally, while an old bur can be employed to bridge larger gaps and Duralay applied to connect it to the copings at either end.

The impression tray is now taken and carefully placed over the connected copings, ensuring that it does not engage any coping or connecting material. The tray can then be removed, loaded with impression paste, and seated carefully over the coping assembly. Each of the coping screws must be undone before the

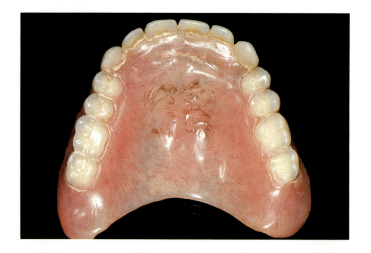

Fig. 7.35. The imprint of lower incisors on the thin palate of a complete upper denture is a danger sign to be taken seriously. A modified impression technique is recommended to provide versatility with abutment selection.

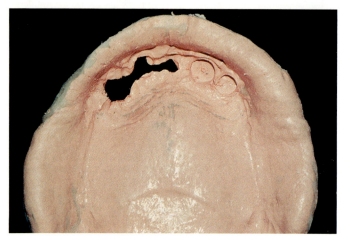

Fig. 7.36 A diagnostic impression made with the healing abutments in place. A window has been cut to allow for the impression copings that will be positioned later.

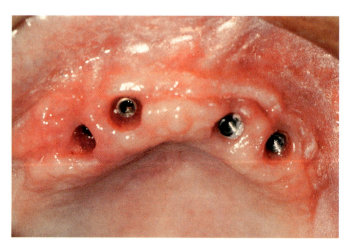

Fig. 7.37. Removal of the healing abutments.

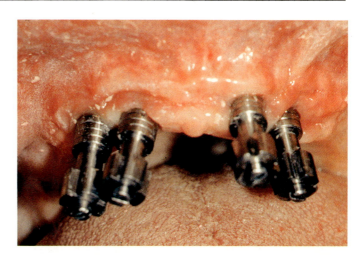

Fig. 7.38. Single tooth impression copings engaging the hexagonal projections of the underlying implants.

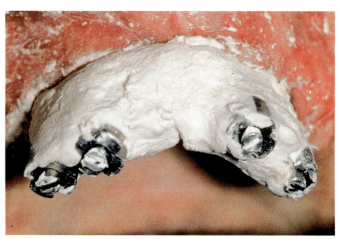

Fig. 7.39. These single tooth impression copings are now locked together with impression plaster.

impression is removed and the healing abutments replaced.

Implant analogues are now attached to the copings and incorporated in the master cast. The bases for jaw relations and trial insertions are constructed on this master cast. If healing abutments, corresponding with those in the mouth, are screwed into the master cast, the wax bases can be adapted to them. This obviates the need to remove the healing abutments from the mouth at subsequent visits for jaw relation recordings and trial locations, while the presence of the healing abutments helps stabilise the bases.

Once the trial insertion has established the position of the artificial teeth, the most appropriate abutments can be selected and design of the superstructure and of the overdenture can be undertaken (Figs. 7.40–7.42). Metal occluding stops on

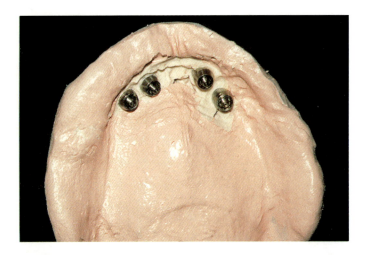

Fig. 7.40. Master impression, incorporating the connected impression copings. The coping assembly has been unscrewed before removal of the impression.

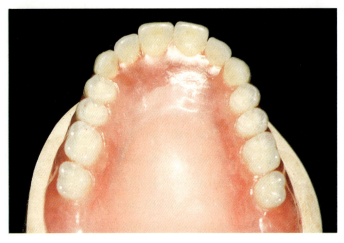

Fig. 7.41. Trial insertion.

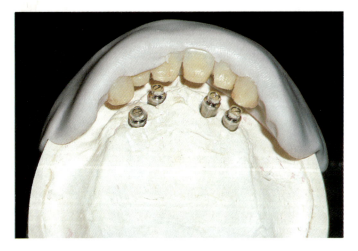

Fig. 7.42. With the aid of a silicone mask, the artificial teeth are held in the same spatial relationship as in the trial insertion. Note that the height of the abutment selected is too great and insufficient room exists for the superstructure. A shorter abutment can now be selected. This versatility would not be possible had a conventional impression over transmucosal abutments been made.

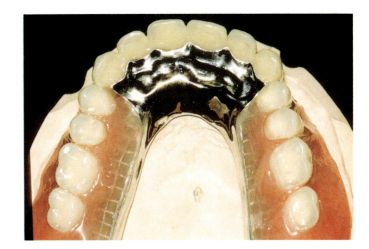

Fig. 7.43. Minimal vertical space is occupied by the metal occluding stops, yet the stiffness of the structure is not compromised.

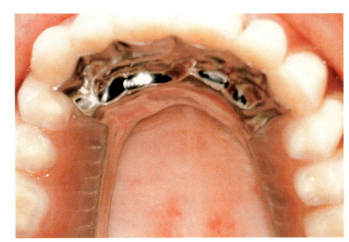

Fig. 7.44. The prosthesis in the mouth.

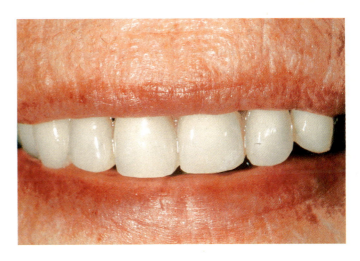

Fig. 7.45. The prosthesis provides adequate lip support.

the overdenture are acceptable and work well; they cannot be incorporated as an afterthought.

Using this approach, unexpected barriers to tooth placement, humps in the palate or bulges in lower overdentures can be avoided. It is a useful route for functional, long-lasting and good looking restorations (Figs. 7.43–7.45).

8 Delivery and post-insertion care

It is often considered that the delivery of the overdenture marks the end of prosthodontic therapy; nothing could be further from the truth. The delivery stage merely marks the end of one phase of treatment and usually indicates that some payment is due. The remaining therapy will take place over many years. Overdentures and their supporting structures require periodic inspection and maintenance, points that should be made clear to the patient at the outset.

The overdentures should arrive from the laboratory complete with remount casts. If these casts have not been provided, undercuts should be blocked out with soft wax and remount casts produced.

Adaptation of bases

The impression surface of the denture must then be carefully inspected for sharp edges or blemishes. Even if none can be seen, the changes that occur during the curing cycle are likely to prevent the acrylic resin being perfectly adapted to all the underlying structures (Fig. 8.1). The adaptation of the base is the first item to be examined, and this step has been simplified by the advent of fast setting silicone based materials such as Fit-Checker. These materials do not easily smear or rub off in the mouth, nor do they clog handpieces: instead they peel away, leaving a clean surface. Such materials may even be used with immediate replacement overdentures. It is possible to tease the disclosing material away from the denture base in one piece, thereby providing the operator with a three-dimensional representation of the space between supporting structures and the denture base.

Silicone based disclosing materials tend to flow under bar retainers and to remain firmly secured to them. The first check for adaptation should be made before the bar retainer has been inserted (Fig. 8.2). Checks later on, or when a duplicate denture is being produced, require that the space under the bar be blocked out. Alternatively, a disclosing paste may be preferred. Once the adaptation of the denture base has been checked,

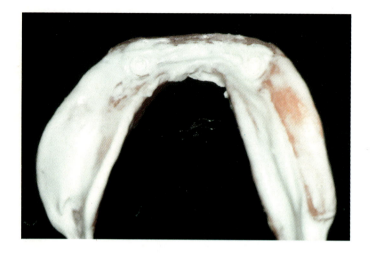

Fig. 8.1. Use of Fit Checker prior to delivery. Note the undue thickness of the labial flange, as well as the areas of excessive pressure.

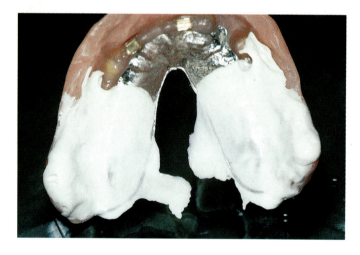

Fig. 8.2. Checking the mucosal borne section of the prosthesis. The material has been kept clear of the bar assembly.

the occlusion and articulation can be examined.

A precise intercuspation of the teeth is essential, but we know that visual examination of the occlusion and articulation provide only a limited idea of what is actually taking place. Even if the teeth appear to intercuspate perfectly, this may well be an illusion caused by small movements of the denture bases on the yielding

mucosa. Furthermore, despite every possible care at the trial insertion stage, there are a number of potential sources of error before the denture reaches the patient's mouth.

These complications are speedily overcome by means of the check record procedure. The entire check record procedure is surprisingly quick and is an excellent investment in time. Visits for subsequent adjust-

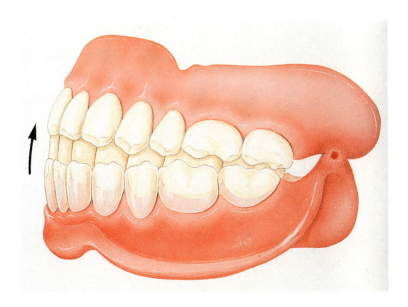

Fig. 8.3. The posterior premature contact may cause direct trauma, while the resultant movement of the denture bases may cause damage elsewhere.

ment are usually reduced, while the patient must benefit from an occlusion and articulation that has been adjusted with precision.

Opposing teeth must not contact during these procedures, otherwise the result of uneven tooth contact may become superimposed on the impression surface of the denture. Fast setting impression plaster is the material of choice for opposing complete dentures (Figs. 8.3–8.11). Where the natural dentition is involved, a wax record is more convenient to employ, although the operator may prefer one of the zinc oxide based recording materials. Silicone based recording media are also eminently suitable.

By carrying out the check record at this stage, two sources of error have been overcome.

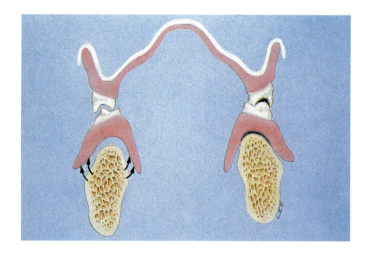

Fig. 8.4. Mucosal displacement may hide small discrepancies. Nevertheless, these errors of jaw relation recording are quite capable of causing damage.

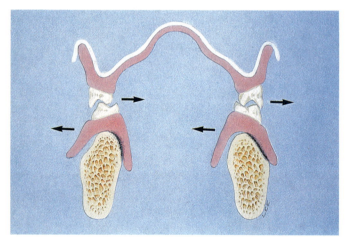

Fig. 8.5. Deflective contacts are difficult to see in the mouth and may cause damage to the areas heavily lined.

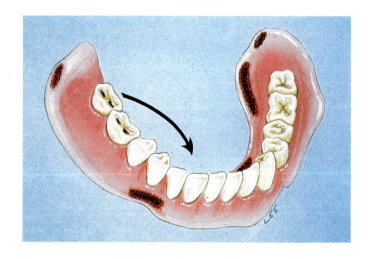

Fig. 8.6. Combined premature and deflective contacts may cause the dentures to rotate, resulting in complex patterns of trauma.

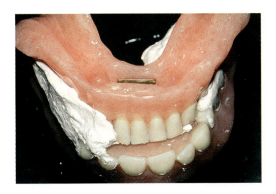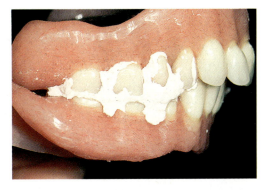

Fig. 8.7 Fast setting impression plaster has been used as the check record material although quick setting silicone materials also produce good results. If possible, remove both dentures together locked by the record.

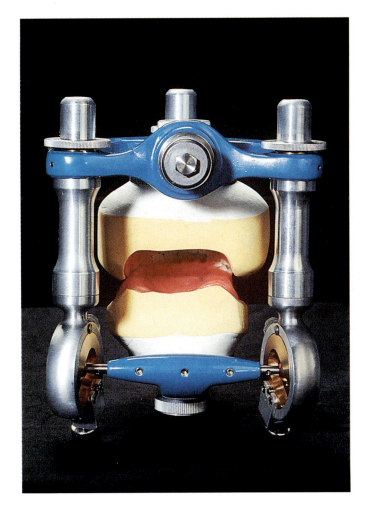

Fig. 8.8. A pneumatically controlled Dentatus articulator is particularly useful for rapid remount procedures.

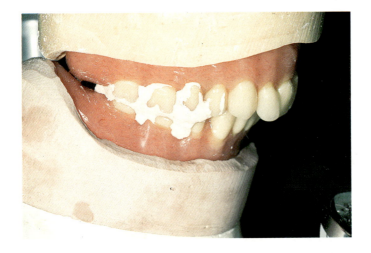

Fig. 8.9. The dentures are now remounted on the articulator.

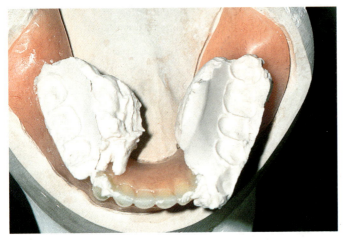

Fig. 8.10. Separation of the dentures.

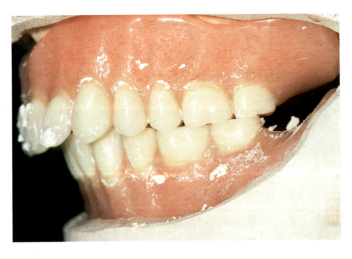

Fig. 8.11. Following removal of the record, corrections to the articulation are straight-forward.

Curing changes

Errors of processing technique may produce very considerable changes in the artificial occlusal surfaces. While the larger errors are generally avoidable, some small movement will inevitably occur during the curing of the denture bases, and the subsequent flasking and polishing. These errors become more noticeable following removal of the dentures from their casts. It is true that the majority of processing changes can be eliminated by using a simple remount technique onto an occlusal index that was made at the trial insertion stage. However, processing changes are only one of the problems with which we are faced.

Clinical errors

The check record is best carried out when the processed dentures are first placed in the patient's mouth. The adaptation of the denture base to its supporting structures will have been checked with a disclosing material. As it is likely that the dentures were processed on the master cast, a new facebow will be required followed by an interocclusal record of centric relation made with the vertical relation increased sufficiently to prevent cuspal contact or interference. The record itself may be made of plaster, wax, or one of the occlusal indicating compounds. The interocclusal record should be kept as thin as possible, consistent with these aims. Fast setting artificial stone, or impression plaster, is a particularly useful medium. By means of the record, the dentures are now remounted on the articulator, the record removed and the occlusion examined with the dentures mounted on unyielding plaster casts. It is then possible to see small errors that would otherwise be masked in the mouth. Articulating paper may be used to mark contact points and there is no danger of smearing due to sliding contacts. It is wise practice to re-record condylar angles and recheck eccentric articulation.

Post-insertion care

Careful explanations throughout the prosthodontic therapy go a long way to helping with post-insertion care and ensuring the patient's co-operation. Following insertion of the overdenture, the patient is advised not to remove it until his adjustment visit the next day. The overdenture is then adjusted in the usual manner using a disclosing material.

At this stage the patient is given further instruction in cleaning his prosthesis and is shown how to brush it with a soft bristle toothbrush and ordinary hand soap. The patient is warned not to use harsh abrasives. It is only at the end of the first postoperative week that the patient is instructed to remove the overdenture at night; he is also told to remove it after each meal if possible and brush it. Disclosing tablets are very useful to demonstrate areas of retained plaque on the denture and the patient is normally given a small supply for this purpose.

For root supported overdentures investigations by Shannon (1980) have shown the value of a water free 0.4% stannous fluoride (SF) gel. This was demonstrably superior in its protective properties to all other compounds. Daily home care by the patient includes cleaning the teeth and gingivae in the conventional manner, followed by brushing the gel onto any dentine surfaces. The patient may expectorate but not rinse, thereby prolonging the contact time between gel and root surface. Every morning, the patient fills the indentations over the roots or attachments with a small amount of gel. Nowadays, many of the fluoride containing toothpastes appear to offer a high degree of protection if placed within the indentation of the denture after plaque has been removed from both denture and abutment. The overriding importance of plaque removal must be stressed and the patient needs to appreciate the importance of regular visits for maintenance.

Gold screws for implant supported overdentures

The first step is to place the bar assembly over the transmucosal abutments and to examine the margins of the copings. If the adaptation appears satisfactory, the superstructure is checked for any tendency to rock. The next step in the test for passive fit is to insert and tighten the screw at one end of the construction and to ensure that the coping at the far end remains adapted (Fig. 8.12). The screw is then removed and the step repeated, but this time placing the screw at the opposite end. Only if the assembly passes these various tests can it be said to demonstrate a passive fit, and one can then proceed to insert the prosthesis. It is normally considered wise practice to insert the screws at either end of the assembly and loosely tighten them before inserting any intermediate screws. Tightening is carried out progressively. Nevertheless, some stretching of the screw is likely to occur and it is quite normal to tighten the screw progressively after each maintenance visit for up to 2 weeks.

Continual loosening of a screw is a danger sign. The first step is to remove the entire bar assembly and check the abutment screw (Fig. 8.13). If the gold screw has become loose, it is quite likely that the abutment screw into which it fits will also have become undone. One of the principle reasons for this type of

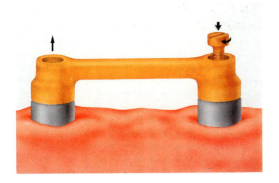 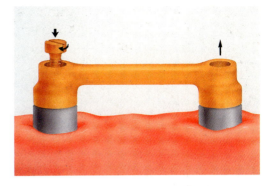

Fig. 8.12. A passive fit can be difficult to achieve. Insert a gold screw at one end of the bar and tighten to see if the other end lifts. Repeat the procedure inserting the screw at the other end first.

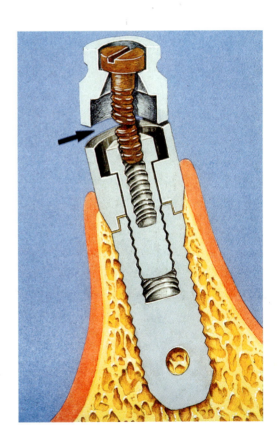

Fig. 8.13. A loose or broken gold screw usually implies a badly fitting gold coping or incorrectly seated abutment.

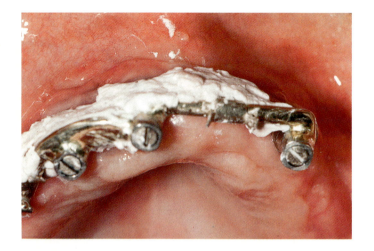

Fig. 8.14. The ill-fitting bar has been cut and the sections relocated with plaster. When cutting the bar, ensure sufficient remains in each segment to allow for accurate relocation.

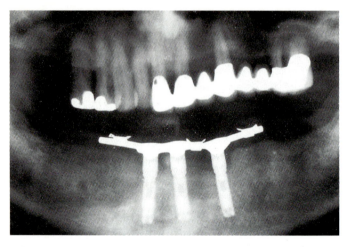

Fig. 8.15. The length of the cantilever and the opposing irregular natural occlusion is likely to lead to fracture of the bar solder joint or damage to the abutment assembly.

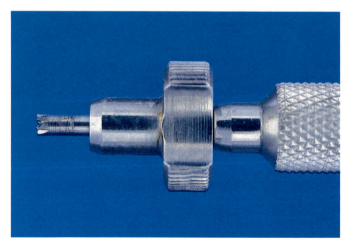

Fig. 8.16. A fractured abutment screw will require removal of the broken tip from within the implant – a difficult task simplified by the special tool provided by the manufacturers.

mishap is that the abutment cylinder was not perfectly seated on the underlying fixture, and although a radiograph should have been taken earlier on, a further one will be required at this stage if there is any doubt in the matter. Should the abutment cylinder not be properly seated, it will need to be removed, any intervening tissue excised and the abutment cylinder reseated and attached for location. It would also be necessary to ensure that the bar assembly fits passively on all the abutment cylinders. If not, it will need to be sectioned, relocated and soldered (Fig. 8.14). Although some clinicians prefer to relocate in the mouth, it is usually simpler to make a new master impression and the entire relocation and subsequent soldering is then all done in the laboratory.

Another cause of continual abutment screw loosening would be excessive loads applied usually to cantilevered extensions on bars (Fig. 8.15). In some circumstances these may lead to fracture of the solder joints, and even fractures of the abutment screw itself are by no means unknown. A fractured abutment screw will require removal of the broken tip from within the implant – a difficult task that is simplified by the special tool available from the manufacturers (Fig. 8.16).

Regular maintenance is vital to the success of any overdenture. Implant supported overdentures appear to be subjected to surprisingly high loads, and provision for regular maintenance is an essential part of treatment planning.

Relining, rebasing and repairs

Relining can be considered to be the process that involves restoring the impression surface of one section of the denture base. Rebasing implies that the entire denture base is involved in the procedure. However, the process is relatively straightforward when an overdenture covers bare root faces of gold copings without attachments, as the procedure is virtually identical to that employed for a complete denture. Even so, the difficulties should not be underestimated, as many a wise clinician has pointed out that rebasing is the easiest technique known for destroying a denture. Alterations are being made both to the impression surface and, inevitably, the occlusal surface as well. It is not a procedure to be undertaken in a hurry, requiring removal of material from the entire impression surface and adaptation of the borders, followed by a careful impression. After processing, a check record is almost certain to be required. However, when attachments are involved the procedure becomes more complicated.

The majority of attachment-retained systems require the retaining element to be buried in the denture base and incorporated within the surrounding acrylic resin. There are one

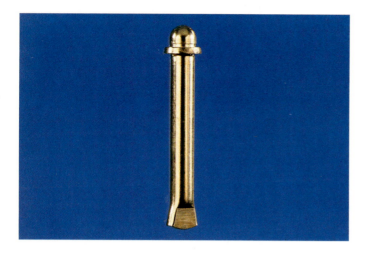

Fig. 8.17. The Dalbo locating dowel for incorporation within the artificial stone of the master cast. This ancillary device is essential for rebasing procedures.

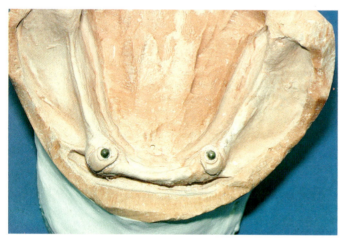

Fig. 8.18. Master cast incorporating Dalbo locating dowels.

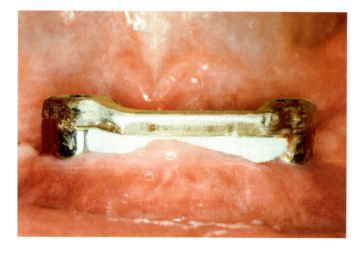

Fig. 8.19. Careful blocking out is essential before any intra-oral relocation of a sleeve is attempted. Any acrylic resin engaging the space under the bar would lock the prosthesis securely in place. Careful blocking out is essential. This blocking out procedure is also used before making an impression for a duplicate denture.

or two notable exceptions. Following relining, rebasing or repair of the acrylic resin, it will be necessary to cure the material, and while this process is occurring it is extremely likely that the attachment will move very slightly within the denture base. The movement may be slight but it will certainly be enough to prevent the denture seating back in the mouth, a mishap that is both time consuming and difficult to repair.

Most manufacturers provide locating dowels to prevent such an unfortunate occurrence. When the impression has been made, the locating dowel is placed over the attachment before the impression is cast so that the locating dowel becomes part of the stone cast on which the denture will be relined or repaired (Fig. 8.17). The locating dowel holds the attachment in its correct position and prevents any possible movement during the curing process (Fig. 8.18). Operators are advised never to attempt these procedures unless they, or their laboratory have in their possession the correct dowels. If movement of the attachment does occur, it will need to be cut out and reincorporated in the denture base using the technique for intra-oral processing that has been described, together with its drawbacks and hazards.

Remaking an attachment-retained denture

With the exception of magnets, virtually all attachments incorporate a depression that will be undercut relative to the path of withdrawal of the denture. If an impression is made in an elastomeric material and cast, it will be difficult to remove the tray and material without damage to the underlying cast. It is true that with bar retainers screwed into place, it is possible to remove the bar and incorporate it in the new master cast, but that leaves the patient without the retainer while the new denture is being produced (Fig. 8.19). Normal practice usually dictates blocking out the space under the bar, including the deepest part of the depression at its base before the impression is made. Little difficulty should be encountered in placing the sleeve or sleeves onto the cast of this impression.

Where stud attachments are concerned metal replicas of the male section of the attachment should be placed in the corresponding depression of the impression before it is cast. These replicas incorporate suitable tagging so that they become part of the master cast.

Troubleshooting

For descriptive purposes maintenance complications can be divided
into:

(a) those involving the removable
    prosthesis;
(b) those involving the fixed struc-
    tures.

The removable prosthesis

In view of the high loads placed on
overdentures, they are particularly
susceptible to errors of jaw relationship leading to overload. Although
articulating paper, judiciously applied, may act as a guide to the
problem, there is no substitute for the
check record and remount procedure. This should be a routine
undertaking before the dentures are
first delivered, but a subsequent
check record is occasionally necessary.

While disclosing pastes such as Fit
Checker are invaluable for checking
adaptation of the denture base, on no
account should the opposing teeth
be allowed to contact while the
material is setting, otherwise the
effects of a possible jaw relation error
may be reproduced on the impression surface. Silicone materials
are clean, easy to assess and fast
setting, but not convenient to use
where bar attachments are employed, as the material flows under
the bar and is left behind when the
removable prosthesis is taken out.

For such restorations, pressure indicating paste should be used.

Any detectable movement of the
denture base under load requires
investigation. Border moulding may
well be required, followed by a
complete rebase. Should the resorption be confined to one section, then
relining this area should suffice and
is to be preferred.

Adjustments of attachments such as
studs and bars need to be undertaken with care, always in stages and
using the manufacturer's instruments when provided. Try to adjust
the retention of the bar by deforming
the entire length of the clip by a small
amount rather than bend a section of
it. Retaining units of nylon, which
cannot be adjusted, will of course
need to be replaced from time to
time. Removal of the old clip and
replacement is quite straightforward.
Broken clips on bar retained overdentures are a common finding on
those supported by implants (Fig.
8.20). While it may be a reflection of
lack of stability of the denture base,
replacing a clip can be a difficult
procedure, apart from the Hader bar
system and similar devices with
easily replaceable nylon clips. In the
case of a small metal clip, such as
the CM Rider, the operator may be
able to drill away the resin from the
small retaining lugs, slide out the
broken clip and insert a replacement
clip into exactly the same space, as
the imprint of the original clip will be
left in the denture base. The very
smallest amount of self-polymerising

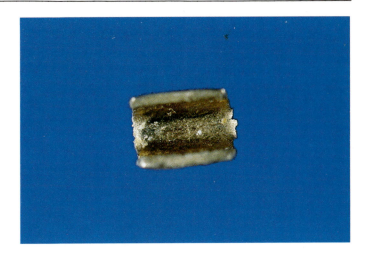

Fig. 8.20. Excessive loads have fractured the tagging from the clip.

resin around the retention lug should be enough to secure it in place and it should be allowed to harden before the denture is replaced in the mouth. If an entire relocation procedure has to be undertaken, a window should be cut into the denture. Never attempt to locate an attachment by placing it in the mouth, filling the denture base with resin and inserting it. The hazards of undertaking a procedure in this way using a bar retainer require little imagination. Even the smallest amount of acrylic resin under the bar will lock the entire restoration securely in place.

Once a window has been cut, the attachment is placed over the corresponding unit in the mouth. Undercuts can be blocked out, preferably with impression plaster, and the denture inserted.

While the denture is held securely in place, the assistant locates the female element of the attachment to the denture base by applying small amounts of self-polymerising resin. No attempt is made to make a complete repair at this stage. Once the acrylic resin has hardened and the location has been shown to be correct, the remaining defects can be filled in by adding increments of acrylic resin which are allowed to polymerise out of the mouth. Once the resin has reached the doughy stage and cannot flow, the denture is placed back into the mouth to ensure that the remaining polymerisation does not cause any change in the relationship of one section of the attachment to the other.

Once in a while the free edge of a metal clip may be bent over by an over zealous patient who then proceeds to attempt to bite the overdenture into place. This type of situation usually presents as an emergency as the denture will not seat. Rescuing the sleeve is a difficult task, requiring care. The edges should be prised gently apart in a

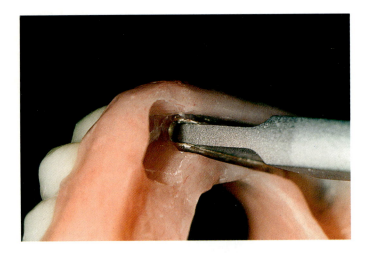

Fig. 8.21. Slackening the Dolder Bar prior to the first insertion of the denture. A special tool is provided.

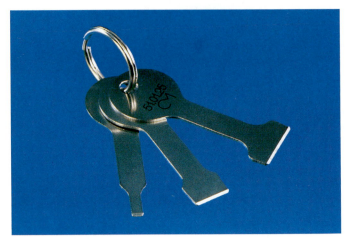

Fig. 8.22. Adjustment tools for increasing the retention of the Dolder Bar joint sleeve.

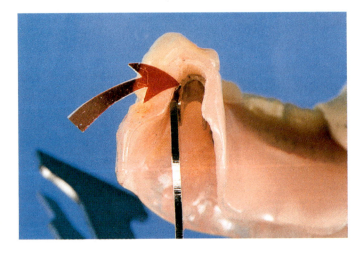

Fig. 8.23. Denture cut away to show method of increasing the retention of the sleeve.

series of stages until it is certain that the prosthesis can be inserted and only then should any attempt be made to provide additional retention. In the case of the Dolder bar, the manufacturers provide a tool that is exactly the same contour as the bar itself and this can be inserted into the sleeve to ensure that it is correctly contoured along its entire length (Figs. 8.21 – 8.23).

Denture base fractures

Repeated fractures of the denture base at a specific point are usually the result of fatigue. Naturally, the first step is to ensure that loads applied to the prosthesis are reduced as much as possible and this in-volves careful checking of the jaw relationship, contours and sizes of the opposing occlusal surfaces. The adaptation of the base should be checked to ensure that there is no tendency for it to rock. Any obvious stress concentrating defects such as "V" shaped notches around frenae will require attention, usually in the form of a fraenoplasty and recontour-ing of the denture flange.

Unfortunately, such repeated frac-tures are often the result of errors in treatment planning that provide in-sufficient bulk of material for the denture base. In these situations the only alternative is to provide more room by remaking the abutment restorations while employing a metal denture base as well.

9 Implant systems and techniques

No matter which type of implant system is employed, an overdenture covering the superstructure acts as a force transfer system of an unpredictable nature. In view of the possible lever arms, the potential for considerable torque application exists.

Implant abutment sites

While the operator may have little choice in the selection of natural abutments, there is far greater versatility when implants are to be employed. Quite often, roots or teeth will be found where the bone support is greatest and the operator will be faced with a decision about whether the site is more valuable than the root that occupies it.

Two implants in the mandible and four implants in the maxilla are the normal minimal requirements. Implant sites, angulation and faciolingual positioning are other important decisions to be made. The importance of bearing in mind the final result right from the initial stage of therapy might be stressed. For example, if a bar and sleeve retainer is planned, it would be pointless to insert four closely spaced implants that make it impossible to find room for a sleeve between them. Such a mishap would necessitate cantilevered distal extensions and the likelihood of the eventual fracture of a soldered joint is increased if there are natural teeth in opposing positions.

Maxillary implant placement and the associated abutments are also more difficult where lower natural teeth are present, due to the limited intermaxillary space that may exist and the problems that will occur if the long axis of the implant impinges against the incisal edge of a lower tooth.

The problems of implant abutments penetrating mobile tissues, of malangulations resulting in eccentric loading, and the aesthetic complications that result from poorly planned implant placement, have all been discussed in other sections of the text. They are mentioned simply to reiterate that the versatility of approach that implants allow the operator brings with it responsibilities of treatment planning and execution that do not arise when natural abutments are employed.

While numerous implant systems now exist, many differing in relatively minor detail, the principles of this book can be applied to most of them. Nevertheless, it was felt helpful to provide a description of three well tried and tested systems.

I am most grateful to Dr. Kristina Arvidson for her contribution on the Astra Tech system and to Dr. Regina Mericske-Stern and Professor Alfred Geering for their section on the I.T.I. approach. These authors have unrivalled experience in their respective fields. No inference, other than space restrictions, should be drawn from the absence in this text of comments upon other implant components.

PART A: The Branemark system

Since much of this text is devoted to the practical applications of the Branemark system, only a brief description of the components will be provided in this section.

Although originally designed for fixed prostheses, the Branemark system has been used to support and retain overdentures for about 15 years. Nowadays, an impressive array of implants is available with diameters of 3 mm, 3.75 mm (standard or self-tapping), 4.0 mm, or 5.00 mm (Fig. 9.1). Implant lengths vary from 7 mm to 20 mm, according to the diameter selected, but the 7 mm length is not recommended for maxillary overdentures. The experimental 3 mm diameter implant is not suitable for overdenture application.

The internal aspect of the implant is protected by a cover screw that remains in place during the phase of integration. It is removed at the second stage when a healing abutment is inserted. One of the most useful modifications of the original Branemark protocol was the introduction of healing abutments. Four heights are produced, 3 mm, 4 mm, 5.5 mm, and 7 mm, according to the soft tissue depth. These are the components that are placed at the second surgical stage and the tissues allowed to heal for about 2 weeks before abutment connection. The transmucosal abutment is now placed by the prosthodontist and the height selected according to the contour of the soft tissues.

The component attached directly to the implant is known as the transmucosal abutment. It is screwed down onto the head of the implant by means of a substantial abutment screw that engages an internal thread within the implant (Fig. 9.2). The design of the implant incorporates a hexagonal projection around the screw hole and this projection is engaged by a matched hexagonal shaped depression in the transmucosal abutment. The differing implants all feature identical hexagonal projections. The engagement of these hexagonal shaped components is critical, and failure to precisely

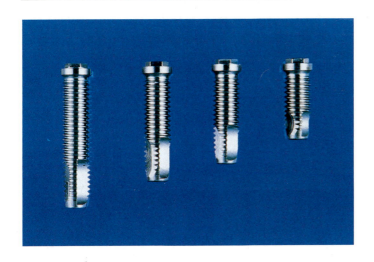

Fig. 9.1. A small selection of the impressive array of implants available with the Branemark system.

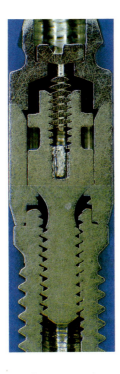

Fig. 9.2. Cross-section of the Branemark system. The transmucosal abutment (TMA) must engage the hexagonal projection of the implant. The TMA is secured by a substantial screw that enters the centre of the implant. Courtesy of R.B. Johns.

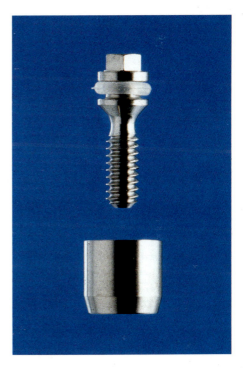

Fig. 9.3. A Branemark transmucosal abutment and matching abutment screw.

191

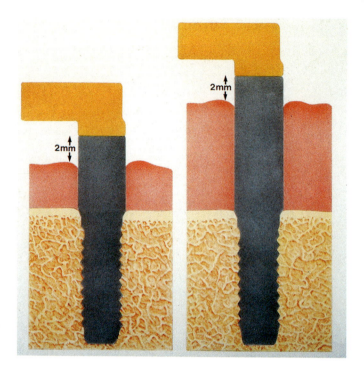

Fig. 9.4. There is considerable leverage potential when a TMA of 8.5 mm or 10 mm is employed.

locate the two components is one of the more common causes of complications.

The transmucosal abutments are available in a variety of heights ranging from 3 mm to 10 mm, depending on the depth of the soft tissue as these abutments need to project some 2 mm above the mucosa (Fig. 9.3). The height of the transmucosal abutment can be judged by the healing abutment that has been employed. The introduction of healing abutments and the modification of the original protocol has gone a long way to improve still further the versatility of the system. If one finds that 8.5 mm or 10 mm transmucosal abutments may be required, the leverage potential should be considered, as the abutment may be approaching the length of the implant before any superstructure is placed upon it (Fig. 9.4). Surgical reduction of the mucosa may provide a better solution in some circumstances.

Since the abutment screw and associated hexagonal interfaces are important components of the force transfer system, not only must the abutment be correctly located upon the implant head but the abutment screw fully tightened to a torque approaching 20 N/cm. If the transmucosal abutment (TMA) is to be left exposed without a superstructure, it should be protected with a titanium

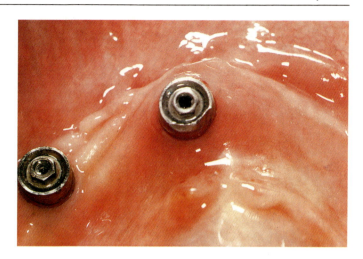

Fig. 9.5. An exposed TMA is easily damaged by an opposing tooth. It should always be protected.

and plastic healing cap as the edges of the abutment are easily burnished or damaged (Fig. 9.5).

The matched impression coping and abutment replica are other important components of the system. The impression coping mirrors the occlusal surface of the transmucosal abutment (Fig. 9.6). It fits precisely over the edges but does not engage the facets of the abutment screw head. The impression coping (and the precious metal coping that will eventually take its place) is therefore free to rotate. It is secured onto the transmucosal abutment by a guide pin that passes through the coping and engages the internal thread within the abutment screw. Guide pins are available in a variety of lengths of up to 20 mm. Where opposing teeth limit the vertical space, a pin flush with the head of the coping is selected, otherwise it is normally considered wise practice to select the longest pin permitted by the available space. Two designs of impression coping are available. The square variety that is removed in the impression is normally the method of choice.

Using a tapered coping that remains in the mouth when the impression is withdrawn may result in potential inaccuracies when the coping is subsequently repositioned in the impression (Fig. 9.7). However, this method does allow the abutment replica and coping to be united out of the impression, so that these two components can be seen to be precisely located before they are placed in the impression.

The other important part of the impression system is the stainless steel abutment replicas. This abutment replica reproduces the occlusal section of the transmucosal abutment, although the facets of the abutment screw head are represented by a cylindrical reproduction (Fig. 9.8).

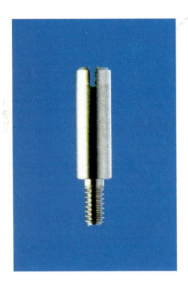

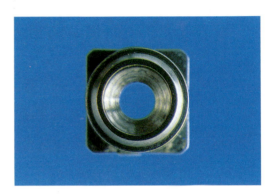

Fig. 9.6. The squared impression coping mirrors the occlusal surface of the transmucosal abutment. It fits precisely over the edges but does not engage the facets of the abutment screw head. Differing lengths of guide pins are available. This coping is removed in the impression.

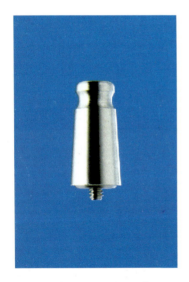

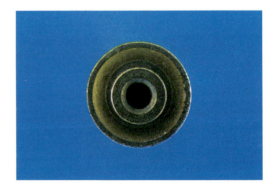

Fig. 9.7. A tapered coping remains in the mouth when the impression is withdrawn. The coping is subsequently repositioned in the impression. Although not normally the method of choice, it may be useful where access is difficult.

Fig. 9.8. The abutment replica reproduces the occlusal section of the transmucosal abutment. The facets of the abutment screw head are represented by a cylindrical reproduction.

Fig. 9.9. Impression copings can be used to stabilise the occlusal rims for jaw relation records. Always use the shortest guide pins.

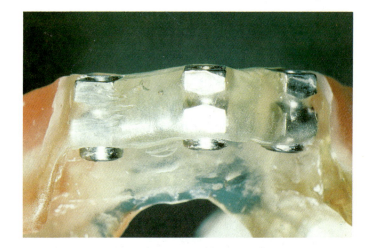

Fig. 9.9.(a)

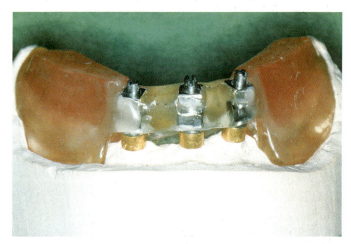

Fig. 9.9.(b)

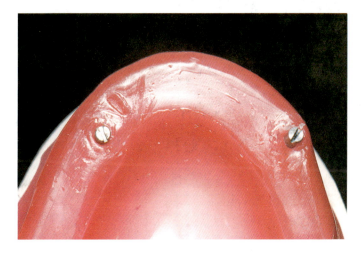

Fig. 9.9.(c)

For most patients, the operator will be making an impression over the transmucosal abutments (Fig. 9.9). The first and essential step is to ensure that these abutments are correctly located on their respective implants, and radiographic confirmation is essential.

Most implant techniques are based on employing the manufacturer's transfer coping which is placed over the transmucosal abutment and secured with a screw. Accuracy can then be assured, provided that there is no intervening debris. In rare situations such as unusual implant angulation, it may be necessary to record the location of the actual head of the implant itself, using a specially produced transfer coping for this purpose. This will be discussed later. A primary impression using alginate in a stock tray is made. A complication here is the adaptation of the stock tray, as the healing abutments will prevent complete seating of the stock tray. If the discrepancy is small, the problem may be overcome using soft wax to border mould the tray, accepting the minor distortion of the sulci that must inevitably occur. Where the projection above the mucosa is larger, the operator will be obliged to use a tray designed for the dentate mouth. In these circumstances distortion of the sulci must occur, and the tray produced on the cast will require extensive border moulding. A modification of the technique is to place tapered impression copings on the abutments before the alginate impression is made. This provides the technician with precise details for the window in the laboratory produced tray.

In constructing the laboratory produced tray, the operator has to provide a window sufficiently large to accommodate the trans-mucosal abutment and the impression coping. Additional spacing should be provided, as the impression copings may be located to one another with a material such as Duralay which may interfere with seating the impression tray unless provision has been made for it. Where implants have been closely opposed, one window is normally made and the location between the transfer copings assured with Duralay applied in small increments. Where widely spaced implants have been placed, the tray is made with two holes through which the transfer copings project. The location between the two copings is assured after the overall impression has been made. Fast setting impression plaster is normally the most convenient, although Duralay can be employed, bearing in mind that the setting time is likely to be greatly increased if placed over a zinc oxide–eugenol type impression paste. Either way, the dental surgery assistant will need to apply additional material over the copings to ensure that they are firmly united. The relationship of the copings to one another is critical and leaves no room for error. A new device to assist in preserving this relationship holds considerable promise. In practice, the actual location of the copings is undertaken once the accuracy of the acrylic resin tray has been assured. Since the impression procedure is time consuming, the use of a diagnostic impression in the custom tray before the placement of transfer copings is strongly recommended. On the basis of the diagnostic impression, the operator can make adjustments to the tray and be assured that when the definitive impression is actually made there is a very good chance that it will be acceptable. The diagnostic impression should be made, the tray adapted, and then cleaned before the transfer copings are placed in the mouth. Since titanium is relatively soft and easily damaged or burnished by opposing teeth or even a denture, healing caps should always be placed over the transmucosal abutments and only removed for the impression procedure.

At least three lengths of screw are available to secure impression copings onto the transmucosal abutment. In the case of the Branemark system the screws, sometimes called guide pins, are 10 mm, 15 mm, and 20 mm long, the shortest being virtually flush with the top of the coping. The longer the screw, the further it will project through the further it will project through the impression tray and the easier it is to loosen after the impression material has been set. The drawback is that the impression tray has to be

manipulated over the screw before it can be seated in place, and so the screw length is selected according to the amount of space available. The shortest screws may well be required in the case of maxillary overdentures opposing natural teeth. In these instances one should take every precaution to ensure that the heads of the screws are easily found and not buried under a mass of impression material, as it is impossible to remove the impression tray until all the screws have been completely loosened. Attempting to remove the impression tray with one screw only partly loosened can be painful and cause damage. Always ensure that the screw is undone. This can be achieved by pulling on the screw head with tweezers to make certain that movement is possible. If the head of the screw is surrounded by impression material or access is difficult, one should continue to unscrew the pin until a pronounced click is felt. Continue unscrewing until the click is repeated. This should ensure that coping and abutment are truly separated.

Once the impression has been removed from the mouth, an analogue representing the transmucosal abutment is carefully placed over the transfer coping. If impression plaster has been used for locating purposes, this may require the analogue to be placed, removed and any loose plaster blown away before it is finally seated on to the impression coping and the screw tightened. Each of the

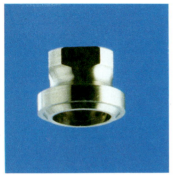 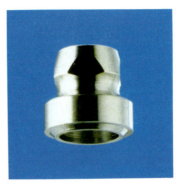

Fig. 9.10. Two heights of gold coping are available, 3 mm and 4 mm. Always use the largest for which space is available.

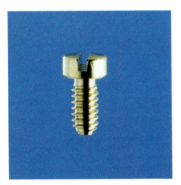 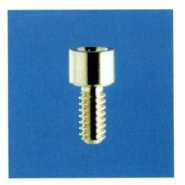

Fig. 9.11. Two designs of gold screw are available to secure the gold coping. The simple slot (left) can be used for either coping, the hexagonal model requires the 4 mm coping.

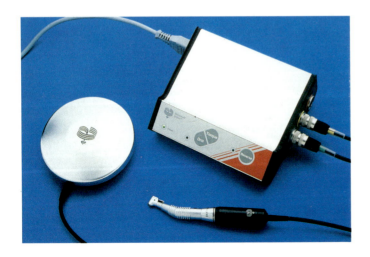

Fig. 9.12. An electronically controlled torque driver is useful to ensure correct tightening of the screw.

abutment replicas is carefully positioned in this manner before the impression is cast. It is normally wise practice for the operator to carry out this procedure in case one of the transfer copings is not adequately secured within the impression. This will be discovered as the screw that unites the coping and the analogue is tightened, and the impression can be remade at the same appointment. Impression copings can be used to produce stabilised wax rims for jaw relation records.

The basis of the superstructure is the gold coping that seats on the transmucosal abutment. It is secured with a gold screw 1.1 mm in diameter. For the standard abutments gold copings of 3 mm or 4 mm height are available, the taller one normally being selected where space permits as it provides a larger surface area for soldering (Fig. 9.10). Two screw head designs are produced, incorporating either a slot or an internal hexagon. Since the head of the hexagon design has to be taller and cannot be used with the shorter coping, the slot is more popular as it assists with standardisation. The gold screw should be tightened to a torque of about 10 Ncm (Fig. 9.11). Other important components to the system include matched screwdrivers and an electronically controlled torque driver (Fig. 9.12).

A stud-type retainer is now produced that replaces the transmucosal abutment (Fig. 9.13). The base of the stud is the abutment screw that engages the centre of the implant. The female component is incorporated in the denture in the conventional manner. Angled abutments are normally best avoided. They complicate plaque control and construction of the prosthesis, and may possibly lead to stress concentrations. However, sometimes their use is inevitable (Fig. 9.14).

Manufacturers normally recommend that the angled transmucosal abutment is placed in the mouth over the implant concerned. A radiograph is essential to make sure it is correctly seated. Angled abutments require special conical shaped healing caps and impression copings (Fig. 9.15). A conical stainless steel analogue is also part of the system. For practical purposes, the impression procedures are identical to those with conventional abutments, apart from the special components. Later on, when the metalwork is constructed, a matching conical shaped precious metal cap is available. This method is very straightforward to use, the only drawback being that the operator has to decide, in the mouth, the exact angulation required, and select the correct height of abutment where a choice is available. Since the abutment may be rotated and secured in one of 12 positions, and there may be more than one angled abutment involved, it is not always easy to make the correct decision at the chairside. Securing the angled abutment with a guide pin can be helpful in this respect.

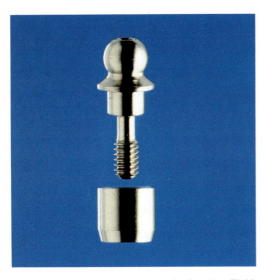

Fig. 9.13. A stud retainer replacing the TMA is now available.

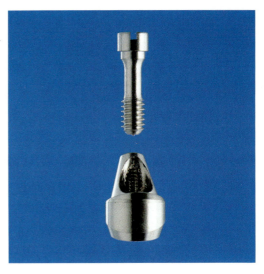

Fig. 9.14. Angled abutments may have to be employed in difficult circumstances.

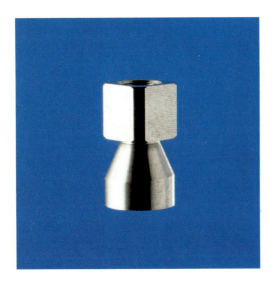

Fig 9.15. Impression coping for angled abutment.

When faced with angled abutments, many experienced operators would prefer to position the abutments in the laboratory. The alignment can be assessed with the aid of a surveyor and the relationship of the abutment together with its superstructure checked against the position of the artificial teeth. These are very considerable advantages well worth the additional clinical complexity.

The first step requires an impression of the implant head, not the transmucosal abutment, and a specially produced transfer coping that fits over the head is required (Fig. 9.15). With the Branemark system this coping incorporates a hexagonal depression to fit over the corresponding projection of the implant.

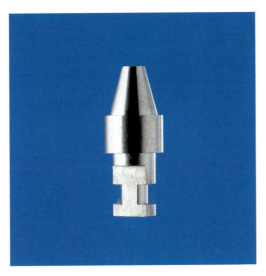

Fig. 9.16. Analogue for angled abutment.

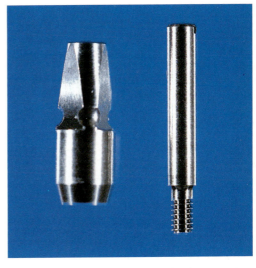

Fig. 9.17. The single tooth impression coping records the head of the implant not the TMA.

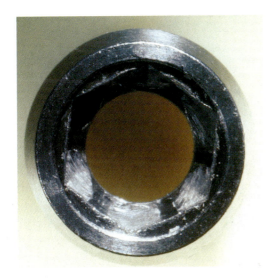

Fig. 9.18. The hexagonal depression must engage the corresponding facets of the projection of the implant head.

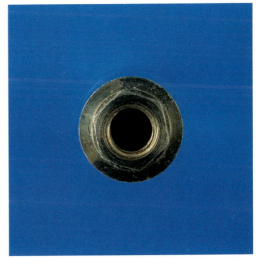

Fig. 9.19. The implant analogue. Note that the hexagonal projection is reproduced.

Graduations on the coping help assess the depth of the implant beneath the mucosa, although this measurement can be obtained from the master cast. Since the adaptation of the transfer coping to the implant is critical and cannot be examined visually, a radiograph must be taken to ensure that it is correctly seated. The transfer coping is incorporated within the impression in the normal manner, but a specially manufactured implant analogue has to be employed representing the head of the implant rather than the transmucosal abutment. A soft material is normally poured around the transfer coping before the impression is cast, but this is not absolutely essential (Figs. 9.16–9.19).

When the impression has been cast, the operator then has in his possession a replica of the patient's jaw incorporating the head of the implant. Jaw relation records and trial insertion procedures are undertaken with this cast, so that the ideal tooth position can be established. A silicone mask is prepared so that the position of the teeth is recorded and the abutments can then be placed on the implant analogues in the best possible relationship. Attempting to complete the superstructure before the trial insertion is a dangerous gamble when angled abutments are necessary. The drawback with this method is that the operator eventually has to place the angled abutment in the mouth in this same relationship, and a small mark to act as a reference point is a great help in this respect. When more than one angled abutment is employed, a resin superstructure is constructed on the master cast, locking the abutments together in their correct relationship. This resin structure incorporates holes to provide access to the abutment screws. The abutment assembly and other components can now be sterilised. The abutments are then carried into the patient's mouth and secured to the resin superstructure. The abutment screws are gradually tightened, moving from one screw to another using not more than three turns at a time, to ensure that the abutments are not pulled out of the resin clamp. In this way, the angled abutments can be positioned in their respective implants in their correct relationship to one another and final tightening of the abutment screws accomplished in the normal manner. Correct seating should be confirmed by means of a radiograph. The versatility and track record of the Branemark system is remarkable. In skilled hands long lasting, functional, and good looking overdentures can be attached to these components with a predictably high success rate. For this to be achieved, the system must be understood together with its limitations.

PART B: The Astra Tech Dental Implant System

Contributed by
Kristina Arvidson
Karolinska Institutet
Stockholm, Sweden

Since 1985, the Astra Tech Dental Implant System has been used in prospective studies at three different university clinics (Arvidson et al. 1992; Gotfredsen et al. 1993); Walmsley et al. 1993). The results to date are promising with regard to scientific, clinical and radiographic parameters. No marked bone resorption has been observed during the first year compared to the 2 subsequent years (Arvidson et al. 1992). However, long-term observations are necessary for definitive conclusions in terms of the criteria for success according to Smith and Zarb in 1989.

Implant components

The Astra Tech Implant is a two-stage titanium implant consisting of a fixture and an abutment. The fixture is a self-tapping screw with parallel sides, which simplifies installation and minimises surgical stress to the bone (Fig. 9.20). The fixture is available in two diameters, 3.5 and 4.0 mm, and in seven lengths, from 8 to 19 mm. The cover screws, placed during the healing period, are also available in two diameters. The abutments, which are self-locating

and self-securing, are designed with a 20 or 45 degree tapered top and are available in six lengths, ranging from minimal height to 7.5 mm, as measured along the parallel-sided neck (Fig. 9.21). An angled abutment is also available, as well as a healing abutment to be replaced as soon as the soft tissue is stabilised after the surgical procedure. The interface between the abutment and the fixture is mediated via a conical seal design that imparts strength and stability to the system and allows self-guiding connection of the abutment to the fixture (Fig. 9.22). The correct seating of the abutment is easily determined, without the need for intra-oral radiographs (Fig. 9.23). The precise-fitting, sealed relationship between the abutment and the fixture, and between the abutment and the prosthetic construction, is reflected in the excellent clinical, radiographic, and histological condition of the soft tissues surrounding the implants (Arvidson et al. 1990, 1992, 1994).

Implantation procedures

Before the implantation procedure, the patients are examined clinically and radiographically as described elsewhere (Arvidson et al. 1992), and the indications for implant treatment must be fulfilled.

The surgical procedure is conducted in two stages. Fixture placement is carried out with the patient under

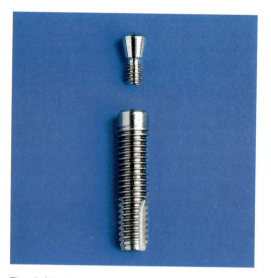

Fig. 9.20. An Astra Tech fixture and a cover screw.

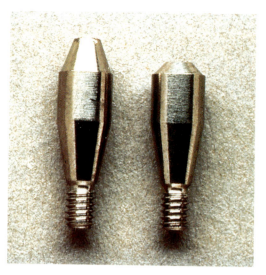

Fig. 9.21. Two uni-abutments with the same 3.0 mm cuff length but with different tapers; abutment 20° to the left and abutment 45° to the right.

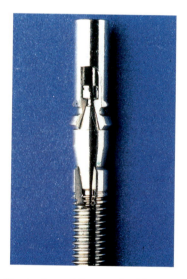

Fig. 9.22. An illustration of the conical interface between the abutment and the fixture, and between the abutment and the restoration.

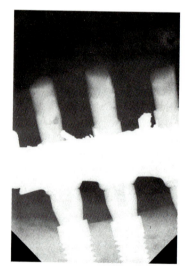

Fig. 9.23. A radiograph of the Astra Tech implant system; fixture, abutment and bridge.

local anaesthesia, in an aseptic environment. Patients are routinely given antibiotic prophylaxis, 1 g phenoximethyl-penicillin twice a day, immediately before surgery and continuing for 1 week postoperatively. After anaesthesia, an alveolar crest incision is made with buccal and lingual mucoperiosteal flap elevation and tissue dissection to identify the bone and the nerve structures. The relative position of the fixture sites is established using a guide drill to perforate the cortical bone. This also allows evaluation of the quality of cortical and cancellous bone. During this procedure preoperative clinical and radiographic evaluations play an important role.

The implant sites are then prepared in a step-by-step procedure using drills of different diameters with indicators giving a direct reading of the correct depth. All preparation of the bone tissue is carried out under copious irrigation with saline at room temperature and with intermittent drilling to prevent heating of bone. Before the fixture is selected, the depth of the implant bed is checked with a depth gauge. The fixture is handled and installed by means of the fixture adapter. The adapter with its mounted fixture can be primarily installed manually or attached to the handpiece connector and handled directly with the contra-angle. The installation is carried out at low speed, 20 rpm, under profuse irrigation with saline at room temperature. Final levelling of the fixture is

done with a ratchet wrench. It is preferable to position the fixture at or slightly below the marginal bone level. Before reposition of the muco-periosteal flaps with interrupted mattress sutures, the cover screws are inserted into the fixtures.

In the upper jaw it is advisable to allow the patient to use the removable upper denture, after some adjustments immediately after the surgery, to limit haematoma formation and swelling. In the lower jaw the old denture is relieved from any compression over the fixture areas, relined and delivered to the patient after 1 week.

The healing period for osseointegration follows generally accepted principles: a minimum of 3 months in the mandible and at least 6 months in the maxilla is advocated. The patient is checked regularly during the healing phase.

The abutment connection is carried out after infiltration or topical application of local anaesthetic. The conical seal design has a strong impact on this procedure. A small incision to confirm the position of the cover screws or a punch instrument is used to remove the overlying mucosa.

Three choices of abutment are available: healing abutment, regular uni-abutment (20°, 45°) or angled abutment. Suitable abutments are selected, mounted on the abutment adapter and installed. Immediately thereafter, the old dentures can be corrected and given a new soft

relining. Based on the angle abutments, the retention of the dentures is usually excellent.

Prosthetic alternatives

The choice of prosthetic alternatives is very much dependent on the degree of resorption. The Astra Tech Dental Implant System has been developed to meet various clinical situations and provide solutions for different prosthetic problems. One of the objectives in developing the system has been to limit the number of components and still provide maximum flexibility with high quality. For an edentulous jaw, the treatment alternatives available, a fixed detachable bridge is often preferable when there are no financial constraints. For the fixed detachable bridge, a good functional, aesthetic and phonetic result depends on a relatively well preserved alveolar process. If there is only limited bone available, the ridge can be augmented successfully in different ways, to provide the desired fixture support and also to improve the phonetic and aesthetic outcome. A less dramatic, yet still beneficial alternative is to provide the patient with an overdenture. This prosthesis has soft-tissue support and does not rely solely on the fixtures for stability.

Overdentures

When using the Astra Tech Implant System, there are four ways of retaining an overdenture; to unite the fixtures via an overdenture bar, or by the use of separate fixtures with special balls or magnets:

- milled bar
- cast bar
- ball
- magnet

No definite contraindications to overdenture treatment have been reported. It should be noted that a minimum of two implants at least 10 mm long is required to support the overdenture.

Treatment planning is based on clinical and radiographical analyses which provide information on optimal bone support at the same time as functional, aesthetic and hygienic requirements are considered. Optimising the temporary removable denture gives an idea of the teeth in relation to the ridge and also the relationship between the teeth.

Plaster or a high viscosity elastic impression material is recommended for the prosthodontic impression procedures, together when using squared impression copings. Plaster (Kühn's impression plaster material) works well for totally edentulous cases with no undercuts. The overdenture cases demand an elastic material and a rigid tray. An individual tray is often made from cold-cure acrylic. Separate holes are made in

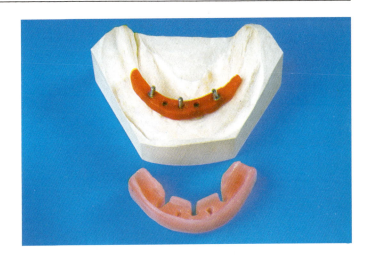

Fig. 9.24. A fixed acrylic resin base and a removable wax rim for registration.

the tray for the penetration of the squared impression copings placed onto the abutments and tightened with the guide pins. When the elastic impression material has set, the impression copings can be further fixed to the tray by using a pattern resin. The tray is separated from the jaw and the impression is inspected. Abutment replicas are placed in the impression copings and tightened with the guide pins. For occlusal registration wax trims are used and it is advisable to use a removable rim as illustrated in Fig. 9.24 on a fixed acrylic record base. With this procedure, it is very easy to check and compare the positions of the abutment replicas on the working cast and the abutments in the jaw.

Well accepted principles of function, aesthetics and patient comfort are the basis for deciding vertical dimension, free-way space, occlusal plane, centric relation, and arch form. If the old denture has been optimised before the implantation treatment, it is very easy to duplicate the old denture and use this duplicate as an impression tray (Figs 9.25–9.27). Security in deciding vertical dimension, occlusal plane, centric relation and arch form, is superior. Further, problems related to adaptation as well as aesthetic and phonetic function can be reduced.

Milled bar

Several concepts have been used for fabrication of overdentures for edentulous patients treated with implants (Engquist et al. 1988). These concepts have all had techniques in common that are known from the treatment of dentate patients and applied to, but not proven suitable for, edentulous patients with implants. Lothigius et al. (1991) have therefore designed a method involving an individually milled or hand-carved

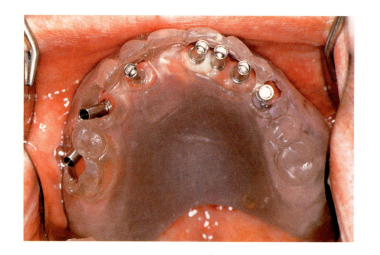

Fig. 9.25. An acrylic resin duplicate of an upper denture used as an impression tray. Both the vertical dimension and the position of the teeth can be transferred to the new tooth set-up.

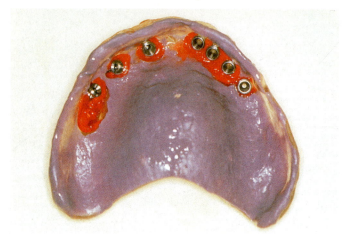

Fig. 9.26. The mucosal view of the duplicate impression. An elastomeric impression material is used to reproduce the mucosa, and the impression copings are attached to the abutments and fixed to the duplicate with resin.

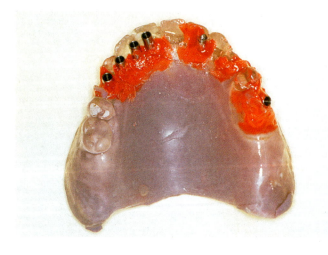

Fig. 9.27. The oral view of the duplicate impression.

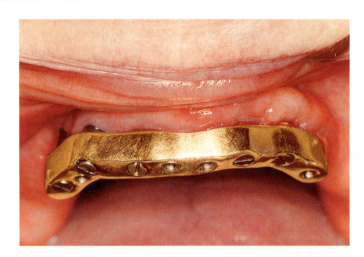

Fig. 9.28. A milled or hand-carved bar splints all implants.

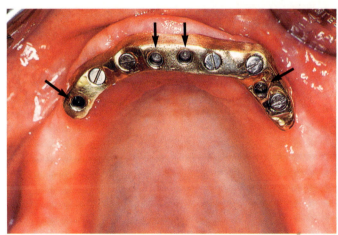

Fig. 9.29. A milled or hand-carved bar splinting four implants; supporting areas on the bar are indicated by arrows. Four Ceka attachments are used. The bar should be positioned immediately behind the labial surface of the teeth to reduce bulk in the restoration.

bar, suitable for two-stage implant systems.

The bar is preferably cast in a type III dental gold alloy and primarily splints the implants (Figs 9.28, 9.29). The bar cross-section should be occlusally converging with an approximately 10° slope to act as a guiding surface. The bar thereby guides the removable structure into place. Distal to the terminal abutments, extensions are made for added lateral stability and support. Three elevated areas on the bar are prepared to give actual support for the overdenture.

The detachable section is a horseshoe-shaped overdenture reinforced by a U-shaped cobalt–chromium (Co-Cr) framework fitting the milled bar and extending over the tuberosities, reinforced and retaining the polymer base material (Fig.9.30). It is recommended that the detachable part of the reconstruction fully cover

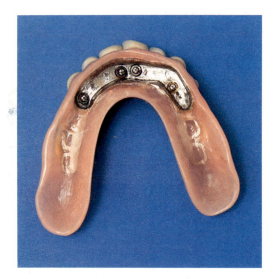

Fig. 9.30. Palatal view of an overdenture retained to a milled bar. Four Ceka attachments are soldered to the framework of Co-Cr. The bar should be positioned immediately behind the lateral surface of the teeth to obtain a less bulky restoration.

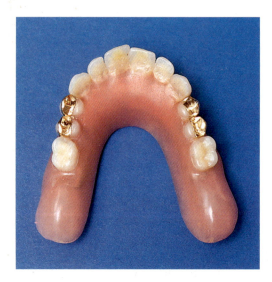

Fig. 9.31. Oral view of an overdenture retained by a milled bar.

the tuberosity to gain maximal support (Fig. 9.31).

The retention between the bar and the overdenture is derived from Ceka Revax attachments (Ceka NY, Antwerp, Belgium). Four attachments are recommended. All female keepers should be kept parallel to one another and to the path of insertion. The removable spring pin, the male part of the attachment, can be placed in the metal framework by either the spacer technique, the soldering technique or the acrylic resin fixation technique (for detailed information see Lothigius et al. 1991).

Cast bar

The implants are connected to a prefabricated/cast alveolar bar and an overdenture is retained with clips (Figs. 9.32–9.35). The overdenture is designed with a maximum denture base, i.e. including a complete denture base. The distance between the supporting implants should not be too great because the rigidity of the bar may be inadequate.

This is a much less expensive procedure for an overdenture than the milled bar. The objective is to position the bar in such a way that retention and stability are achieved with a minimum of torque forces against the fixtures. Gotfredsen et al. (1993) have reported promising clinical and radiographic results for such bar attachment systems attached to Astra Dental Implants for retention of mandibular overdentures.

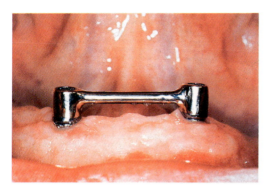

Fig. 9.32. Prefabricated bar retained by two fixtures.

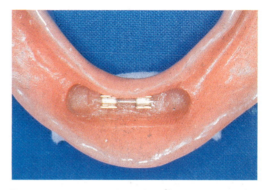

Fig. 9.33. Mucosal view of an overdenture retained to a bar, as illustrated in Fig. 9.31, retained with clips.

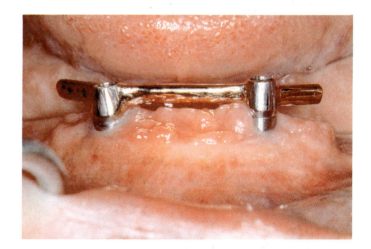

Fig. 9.34. Intermediate and distal bars retained by two fixtures.

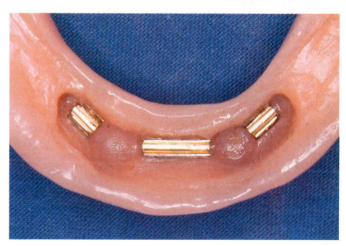

Fig. 9.35. Mucosal view of an overdenture, retained by the construction as shown in Fig. 9.34.

Ball attachment

Individual standing implants with attachments supporting an overdenture are essential in situations where there is a large distance between the fixtures. It should preferably be used in the lower jaw where each fixture has good cortical retention. Even though good bone support is essential in these situations, torque movements and transverse forces against the fixtures must be minimized. With the Astra Tech Ball Attachment (Figs 9.36, 9.37), some rotation and vertical resilience is permitted, thereby relieving the fixtures from unfavourable forces. Gotfredsen et al. (1993) have presented promising preliminary results for ball attachments used as retainers for mandibular overdentures.

Magnet attachment

Basically, the same indications apply for both magnet and ball attachments. A "stress breaking" situation with the magnet attachment reduces the forces acting against the implant. The magnet attachment denture allows some freedom in regard to the path of insertion, even with a rather advanced, non-parallel orientation between the implants (Figs 9.38, 9.39).

The magnet keeper, located on the 45° uni-abutment, is made from a titanium-coated iron-neodynium-boron magnet. It works together with the magnet in a "split-pole" way. Walmsley et al. (1993) have used this technique for retention of overdentures in 20 patients.

Conclusion

Overdentures on implants are usually the treatment of choice when only two or three implant fixtures are installed due to lack of bone or for financial reasons. It is of importance to make as much space as possible for the teeth, base material and the retainers of an overdenture. Therefore 45° top-angled uni-abutments are then preferable to 20°.

In the maxilla, overdentures facilitate the restoration of aesthetics and phonetics and ensure optimal conditions for oral hygiene. Therefore, overdenture therapy in the upper jaw might also be the treatment of choice even when four or more fixtures can be installed. The subsequent lack of lip support may change the facial profile and thus impair aesthetics (Figs 9.40, 9.41).

Maxillary fixed prostheses may also create a problem with phonetics because of an unavoidable space between the residual ridge and tissue side of the restoration. Furthermore, phonetics can be impaired because of a short dental arch, and as implants are sometimes located quite palatally, the irregular bulge of metal around the abutments can obstruct proper phonetics.

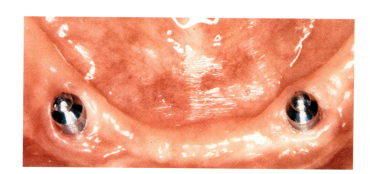

Fig. 9.36. Two ball attachments used for retaining an overdenture attached with O-rings.

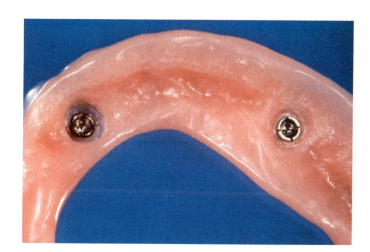

Fig. 9.37. Mucosal view of an overdenture retained by ball attachments.

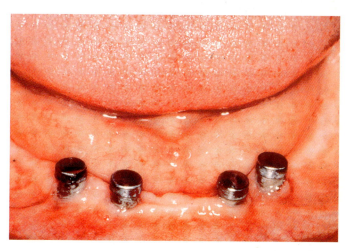

Fig. 9.38. Four abutments with magnet keepers.

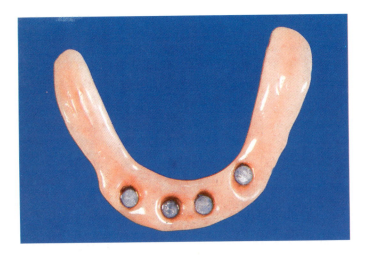

Fig. 9.39. Mucosal view of an overdenture retained by magnet attachments.

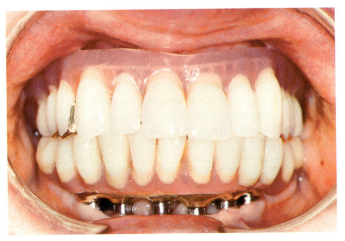

Fig. 9.40. Frontal view of an overdenture on a milled bar in the upper jaw and a bridge in the lower jaw, both retained by Astra Tech dental implants.

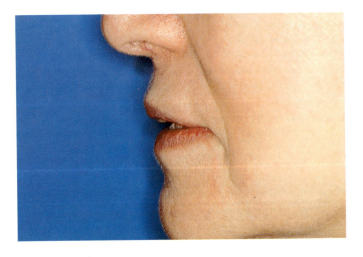

Fig. 9.41. After treatment with an overdenture in the upper jaw and a fixed detachable bridge in the lower jaw, both retained by Astra Tech dental implants.

References

Arvidson K., Bystedt H., Ericsson I. Histo-metric and ultrastructural studies of tissues surrounding Astra Dental Implants in dogs. Int J. Oral Maxillofac. Implants 1990; 5: 127-134

Arvidson K., Bystedt H., Frykholm A., von Konow L., Lothigius E. A 3-year clinical study of Astra Dental Implants in the treatment of edentulous mandibles. Int. J. Oral Maxillofac. Implants 1992; 7: 321-329

Arvidson K., Bystedt H., Frykholm A., von Konow L., Loathigius E. Results from prospective studies with Astra Tech dental implants presented at 72nd Annual Meeting of the IADR, March 9-13, 1994

Engquist B., Bergendal T., Kallus T., Linden U. A retrospective multicenter evaluation of osseointegrated implants supporting overdentures. Int. J. Oral Maxillofac. Implants 1988; 3: 129-134

Gotfredsen K., Holm B., Sewerin I., Harder F., Hjörting-Hansen E., Pedersen C.S., Christensen K. Marginal tissue response adjacent to Astra Dental Implants supporting overdentures in the mandible. A 2-year follow-up study. Clin. Oral Impl. Res. 1993; 4: 83-89

Lothigius E., Smedberg, J.-I., De Buck V., Nilner K. A new design for a hybrid prosthesis supported by osseointegrated implants: Part 1. Technical aspects. Int. J. Oral Maxillofac. Implants 1991; 6: 80-86

Smith D.E., Zarb G.A. Criteria for success of osseointegrated endosseous implants. J. Prosthet. Dent. 1989; 62: 567-572

Walmsley A.D., Brady C.L., Smith P.L., Frame J.W. Magnet retained overdentures using the Astra Dental Implant System. Brit. Dent. J. 1993; 174: 399-404

PART C: The Bonefit ITI System

Contributed by
Regina Mericske-Stern,
Alfred H. Geering
University of Bern, Switzerland

Excellent long term results have been achieved with this versatile system, that lends itself to over-denture applications. Treatment planning and the selection of patients require protocols similar to other systems. Bonefit ITI implants may be inserted in patients of all ages, while the simple surgical requirements may allow them to be employed where other systems are inappro-priate. The elderly are therefore a group to benefit from these implants, provided that proper medical pre-cautions are taken.

Bonefit ITI implants and drilling system

Material

The implants are made of commer-cially pure titanium. The intraos-seous part of all Bonefit ITI implants is coated with a plasma-flame-sprayed layer, whereas the trans-mucosal neck portion is smooth and polished. The microscopic structure of the coating is designed to provide for enlargement of the surface and to enhance bone apposition onto the implants.

Design

The Bonefit ITI implant currently used for overdenture retention is a two-part implant with an open, trans-mucosal design. Therefore, a one-stage surgical approach is required. The two-part implant type appeared to be more advantageous during the healing phase. Three types of two-part Bonefit ITI implants are used: hollow cylinders, hollow screws and solid screws. The screws are not self-tapping. The three lengths are 8, 10 and 12 mm. The solid screws are available with two diameters: 3.4 and 4.1 mm. Different prefabricated abut-ments can be mounted directly on the two-part implants and are used to retain the dentures. Since solid screws became available (1987), they have been regularly used for overdenture support and the drilling system for the screw shaped im-plants is demonstrated and ex-plained in this book (Fig. 9.42 a, b).

Implant delivery and storage

The implants are delivered in single small glass containers with a screw-top. Sterilisation of the glass con-tainers is necessary prior to surgery. This delivery system provides for safe removal of the implant from the glass package during the surgical procedure and for initial insertion into the prepared implant bed. This screw-top is then replaced with a screw driver and the implant is finally threaded into the bone, using a

Fig. 9.42(a). Two-part Bone-fit ITI implants: hollow cylinder (left angulated), hollow screw, full body screw. (b) Surgical procedure step by step (instruments): round bur, twist drills (two diameters), trephine, gauge, screw tap, implant bed, implant *in situ*.

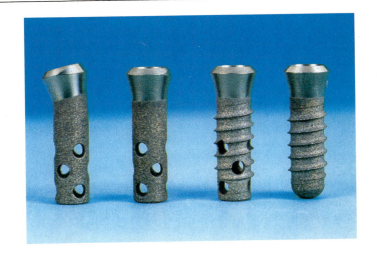

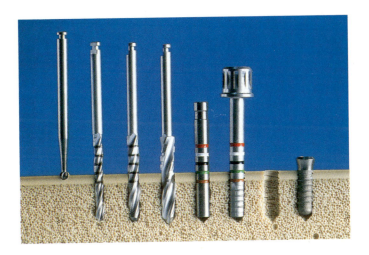

ratchet. Any contact or contamination of the implants with gloves or other materials is avoided. The colour of the screw-top corresponds with the three different lengths of the implants: brown is 8 mm, green is 10 mm, black is 12 mm. Boxes are available to store the glass containers and the surgical instruments.

Drilling system step by step

Round burs with three diameters: to penetrate and open the cortical bone. Twist drills (small and large diameter): to cut the bone and to prepare the implant bed to the desired depth. The diameter is 3.4 mm. The trephine (one diameter): is used to cut the implant bed for implants of a diameter of 4.1 mm.

217

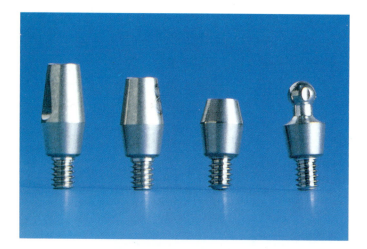

Fig. 9.43(a). Euro system: conical abutments and single stud attachment (right). Second from left: conical abutment (8°) for mounting bars. (b) Octa system: octagonal abutment for placement of crowns and bars.

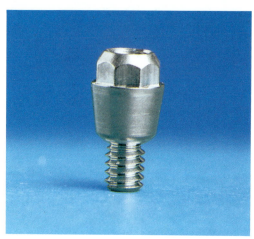

Direction indicators (two diameters): they are used for parallel alignment of the implants and to identify the penetration depth. Screw tap (two diameters): for manual use only, to cut the threads. The screw taps are used with a ratchet. The coloured marks of the direction indicators and the screw taps correspond with the implant length. During the healing phase, cover screws with different designs are selected according to the local, individual situation of the soft tissue.

Attachments used with Bonefit ITI implants for overdenture support (Fig. 9.43 a, b)

Nowadays, two types of attachment are available in combination with two-part ITI implants:

1. Spherical single attachments

(Dalla Bona) are mounted directly on the implants.

2. Implant abutments with a conical-cylindrical (EURO system) or octagonal (US system) design Prefabricated or individually cast gold bars are soldered to prefabricated gold copings that fit exactly to the abutments. The completed bars are connected to the abutments by screws (Fig. 9.44).

Oral diagnosis and treatment planning

The purpose of the presurgical oral diagnosis and treatment planning is:

To determine the number and optimum location of the implants.

To provide for a favourable distribution of the implants over the arch.

To avoid discrepancies between the design of the dentures, implant location and retentive devices, such as bar connectors or single attachments.

The treatment planning protocol includes:

1. clinical oral diagnosis;
2. radiographs;
3. examination of old dentures;
4. number of implants to be placed.

The clinical oral examination

This examination – visual and by palpation – is the first step in order to obtain information about shape, width and height of the residual

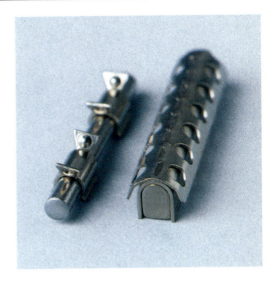

Fig. 9.44. Prefabricated bars: round bar (left), U-shaped bar (right), both with female retainers.

ridges and about soft tissue conditions. Horizontal and vertial relationship of the residual ridges are examined, and space required for the prospective implants and retention devices is evaluated. The fact is that most patients with advanced and severe reduction of the residual ridge are treated with implants. Inadequate space available for placing implants and mounting a bar underneath the denture, is seldom encountered.

Placement of implants within attached keratinised mucosa does not seem to be a prerequisite for the health of the soft tissue, surrounding the implants. According to our own experience and to other published data, attached keratinised mucosa is no longer considered necessary and gingival-mucosal grafting is never prescribed.

Bone mapping of the maxillary ridge may be useful because of the thickness of the palatal mucosa, that disguises the shape of the ridge. It is unnecessary for the mandible. The height of the floor of the mouth in most patients would not allow identification of the shape of the lingual mandibular bone.

Radiographs

Panoramic radiographs are taken of all patients. Checks are made of the sinus and location of the mandibular nerve, bone structure regarding density, pathological findings and presence of residual roots. Bone density is difficult to assess by simple radiographic methods.

A loose structure of trabecular bone without a dense cortical layer, protecting the outer surface of the residual ridge, is mainly encountered in the maxilla. In some cases it is advisable to use the implant screws in the manner of self-tapping screws. In the mandible, dense cortical bone covering the residual ridge, is more often found. In cases with very loose trabecular bone it is advantageous to seek bicortical anchorage of the implants, i.e. of the cervical and apical portion. Clinical experience suggests that osseointegration and remodelling after loading of the implant occurs, even with very loose trabecular bone. However, we do not know the forces of removal torque of these osseointegrated implants.

They would probably be significantly different.

Templates with metallic markers of known diameter allow measurement of the effective bone height and determination of a favourable prospective location of the implants with respect to the topography of the mandibular nerve or maxillary sinus. Cephalometric radiographs give more information about the lingual aspect of the residual mandibular bone and the shape of the maxillary ridge. Exact measurement of width and height are possible, and information about the prospective implant axis in faciolingual dimensions are obtained. For many patients cephalometric radiographs are, therefore, recommended. In our own clinical experience, an advanced degree of atrophy of mandibular ridges was seldom found, and placement of implants with an intraosseous length of 7-8 mm was usually possible. Computer tomograms are not used for the interforaminal placement of two, three or four implants but they can be helpful for treatment planning with maxillary implants (Fig. 9.45a–c).

Examination of old dentures

The evaluation of existing dentures to decide whether they are adequate for temporary use during the healing phase is important. Due to the open healing phase of the Bonefit ITI implants, some difficulties may be encountered projecting them from inadvertent loading. Patients are

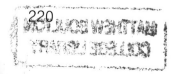

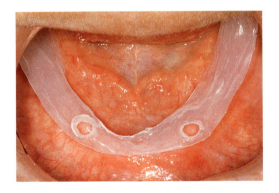

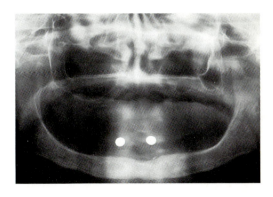

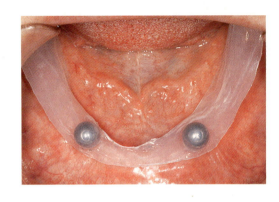

Fig. 9.45 (a). Presurgical evaluation: splint with metallic markers. (b) Orthopanoramic radiograph showing metallic markers. (c) The same splint may be used as a surgical guide.

unwilling to remain without dentures during the whole healing period. If stability of old dentures cannot be provided by occlusal adjustment and relining, new dentures should be made prior to surgery. Old dentures are also examined regarding aesthetics and loss of vertical dimension. Clinical experience shows that many patients, willing to undergo implant surgery because of denture wearing problems, are in need of new dentures. The patients should be told that implants do not compensate for technically and functionally inadequate dentures. Therefore, for many patients the construction of new dentures should precede implant surgery.

Number of implants to be placed

For the support of maxillary overdentures, the placement of three to four implants should be planned. The implants will be connected by a bar.

1. Divergent implant axes, the shape of the ridge and loose trabecular bone are contraindications for the placement of only two maxillary implants.

2. Due to the curvature of the maxillary ridge, short bar segments of 8–12 mm, connecting multiple implants, are suggested. They are more likely to follow the ridge without reducing the palatal space. The space for the tongue will remain free.

For mandibular overdentures, two implants will provide sufficient support for the majority of patients.

1. Straight ridges in the front: the bar connects the two implants in the shortest way – in a straight line. The prospective distance between the central axes of the two implants should be more than 12 mm. This provides for sufficient space to mount female parts. Round bars (non-rigid) or U-shaped bars (rigid retention) may be mounted.

2. Light curvature of the ridge: round bars following the curvature of the ridge may be mounted. The distance between the two implants should allow for the mounting of two female parts. Space required for mounting one female part is approximately 7 mm.

3. Pronounced curvature of the ridge: the placement of three or four implants is suggested. Shorter segments of the bars will not interfere with the profile of the ridge.

Surgical procedure, post-surgical maintenance and healing phases

Premedication

Sedation is usually unnecessary unless patients are very anxious and have a low stress level. The prescription should be made by the physician if the patient is already taking several medications. Antibiotics are given only with diabetes, anticoagulation, irradiated bone, endocarditis, or by recommendation of the physician.

Anaesthesia

Blocks of the mental nerve are unnecessary. Local terminal infiltration with UltracainR containing epinephrine provides for sufficient anaesthesia to complete the entire surgical procedure. Local anaesthetics without epinephrine will not provide sufficient operation time.

Aseptic measures

They must be respected carefully to avoid any contamination of non-infected healthy bone sites. Nevertheless, in order to check temperature and colour of skin, lips, sweat beads and eyes, we do not recommend covering the face (except hair) of the patients with sterile towels, particularly in high risk patients. Well aired rooms with windows may reduce or avoid a claustrophobic feeling.

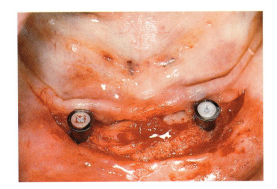

Fig. 9.46. Surgical site: two implants have been placed in the interforaminal area.

Surgery

Surgery should be carried out as quickly and atraumatically as possible, to reduce strain on the patient and on the tissues and to enhance better wound healing. Surgical guides or templates are not regarded necessary for the placement of implants designed to support overdentures, particularly in the mandible when only two implants are to be placed. The preferred position is the location of the canines or slightly more to the midline, and symmetrical to the midline. However, for beginners in implantology, the use of guides and templates may be recommended, they are also recommended in order to check the prospective direction of the implant axis in the maxilla.

The canine area in the edentulous ridge may be located using the dentures worn by the patient. If more than two implants are to be placed – and this is always advised for the maxilla – the implants should be evenly distributed over the segment of the arch, with a minimum separation of 10 mm. This distance provides for a favourable length of the segments of the bar.

After raising the mucoperiosteal flap, the prospective bone sites are checked regarding their width and shape. Then the bone cutting procedures are completed. Whenever possible, bicortical anchorage of the implant is suggested for the mandible. For parallel placement of the implants, the direction indicators are always used (Fig. 9.46). All bone cutting procedures are carried out by cooling with refrigerated saline. Before repositioning of the flap with tight sutures, cover-screws are mounted on the implants.

Post-surgical recommendations

The patient is given effective analgetics for use at home, if needed, although severe post-surgical pains are seldom reported. Intermittent cooling with ice-water is recommended and the patient is informed about diet. Hygiene instructions are given. As the ITI implant has an open

223

transmucosal design, rinsing with chlorhexidine 3 times a day is necessary in the early post-surgical phase.

Healing period

After 7-10 days, depending on the process of wound healing, the sutures are removed. The dentures are provisionally adapted and given to the patient 2-3 weeks after surgery. The denture base has to be relieved above the implants. Soft reliners are used for better adaptation of the denture base to the denture bearing tissue. Stable support of the dentures must be provided by adequate fit in the posterior area of the edentulous ridges. The implants should also be protected from contact with the relined denture base. Furthermore, the patient is instructed about careful use of the dentures. Wearing of temporary dentures during the healing phase may fulfil social and cosmetic demands, but not those of chewing.

Cleaning instructions

During the entire healing period of 3 (mandible) to 6 (maxilla) months, the implant shoulder, surrounded by the soft tissue, has to be cleaned with small multi-tufted brushes. Additional products containing chlorhexidine may be used to facilitate removal of plaque. Maxillary and mandibular dentures have to be removed before sleeping to avoid any parafunctional habits. The soft reliners have to be changed regularly.

Prosthodontic procedures

The connection of complete dentures to osseointegrated implants resembles overdentures retained by natural roots and copings. Receptors of the oral mucosa, the bone, the temporomandibular joints and muscle spindles are involved in coordinating chewing activity in edentulous and dentate subjects, and may substitute for the missing periodontal receptors around implants. It seems that the masticatory stability of overdentures when supported by implants is of greater importance for oral function than the presence of a periodontal ligament itself. Patients with implants are highly satisfied and report a feeling of their own natural teeth. However, there is scientific evidence that the tactile oral sensibility with implant supported overdentures is different from overdentures supported by roots.

Designing implant supported overdentures resembles fundamental principles of constructing complete dentures.

Complete denture approach

The denture design

A complete denture is provided with a well fitting denture base and properly extended flanges. In the case of implant retained overdentures, the denture base should be slightly reduced as soreness of the soft tissue may be caused by the denture flanges due to the relative immobility of the overdenture. Retention of the denture by peripheral seal is not required for overdentures. The replication of lost tissue and the support of facial morphology are provided by the denture base.

Occlusion

Tooth arrangement and selective tooth set-up contribute to retention and stability of the dentures. The (semi) anatomic Condyloform porcelain teeth are used. The occlusal scheme is a tolerant cusp to fossa intercuspidation and bilateral balanced guidance. The arrangement of front teeth allows an anterior horizontal overlap of 1 mm without contact. Despite the lack of scientific evidence, stability of occlusion is likely to be a contributing factor to protect implants from overloading.

Aesthetics

The selection and arrangement of anterior teeth follows basic guidelines for tooth set-up. Individual wishes of the patients can be fulfilled, but should not interfere with fundamental principles of complete denture construction. The set-up of anterior teeth should not interfere with the activity of the perioral muscles.

Clinical and laboratory procedures

Overdentures supported by implants, like their root supported counterparts, require correct load distribution between residual ridge and abutments. The key rests with the impression technique. The preliminary impression is made with metal stock trays and alginate. Individual acrylic resin trays are fabricated with openings for mounting the transfer abutments on the implants. The final impression is made following the altered cast method. The impression of the denture foundation area is made with zinc oxide–eugenol paste. Hard polyether material is administered by a syringe to retain the transfer abutments (Figs. 9.47–9.49). During hardening of the material, the fixation screws of the transfer abutments have to be uncovered and cleaned from all impression materials. After removing the impression from the mouth, the implant analogues are mounted and connected to the transfer copings by means of the fixation-screws, and the master cast is poured. Then the step-by-step procedures of complete denture construction follows. Occlusion wax rims on shellac bases are used to determine the vertical dimension and the level of the occlusal plane, and to record the maxillomandibular relation. The transfer of the intraoral registration to the articulator is always done by using the face bow, indicating the arbitrary hinge axis. After completion of the tooth set-up,

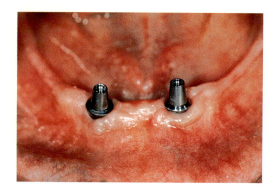 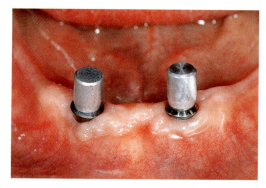

Fig. 9.47.(a) Euro system: 8° conical abutment is mounted. (b) Transfer copings are placed for altered cast impression technique.

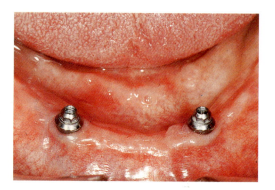 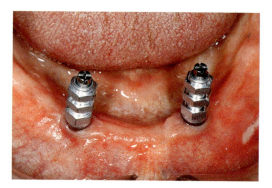

Fig. 9.48.(a) Octa system: octagonal abutment is mounted. (b) Transfer copings are mounted and fixed with screws.

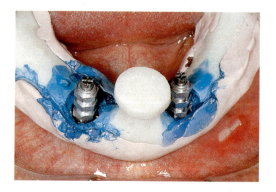 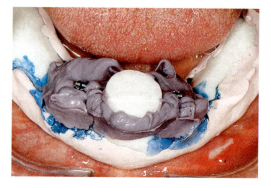

Fig. 9.49.(a) Altered cast impression technique: zinc oxide- eugenol paste for impression of the denture foundation area. (b) Polyether material is applied with a syringe to fix the transfer copings.

226

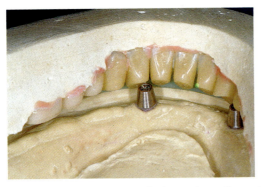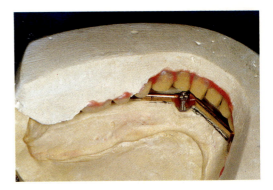

Fig. 9.50.(a) Orientation index of tooth set-up. (b) Bar is fabricated according to the shape of the ridge and with respect to the tooth position of the prospective denture.

the trial dentures in wax are checked with the patient and corrections are made. Following this, the finishing touches to the dentures are processed in the laboratory. For casting the bar, an orientation index of the tooth position is used, that has been taken before the wax is boiled out (Fig. 9.50). Requirements for the placement of the bar are:

1. to follow the shape of the ridge;
2. to respect the position of the artificial teeth;
3. not to reduce the space of the tongue;
4. to provide for accessibility for oral hygiene.

The same orientation index is used to cast the metal framework after final soldering of the bar. The female parts are usually fixed in the denture base during the laboratory procedures, but they can also be mounted directly in the mouth of the patient. They are fixed to the acrylic resin denture base and not soldered to the cast metal framework (Fig. 9.51). If single attach-

ments are planned for retention of the overdenture, these are mounted directly on the implants at the final delivery of the dentures. The female retainers are then polymerised to the denture base in the mouth of the patient.

Support, retention mechanism and retention devices

General aspects of retention and support of overdentures are independent from the implant system that is used. The sum of the retentive strength and support results from various contributing factors:

Number of supporting implants.
Distribution of the implants over the segment of the ridge.
Type and size of the attachments/bars.
Length of the bar or of bar segments.
Number of female retainers.
Degree of atrophy of the residual ridge.

The retention mechanisms of overdentures with Bonefit ITI implants

227

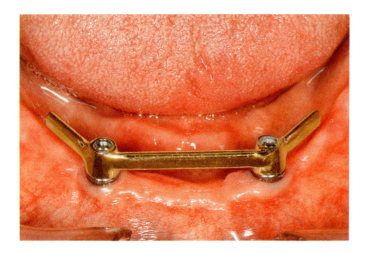

Fig. 9.51 (a). Completed bar: U-shaped bar with distal extensions. (b) Completed denture with cast metal framework. (c) Female retainers mounted in the denture base.

Fig. 9.51.(a)

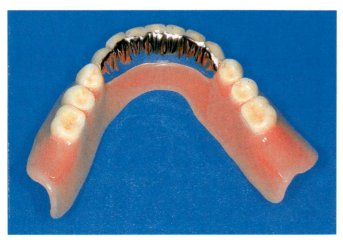

Fig. 9.51.(b)

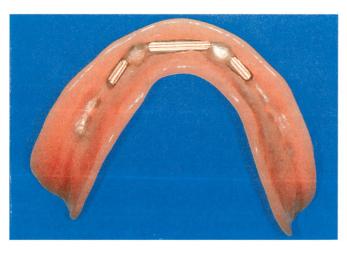

Fig. 9.51.(c)

may be resilient or rigid. The choice of any preferred retention mechanism does not influence the impression technique. The retention mechanism of spherical anchors is resilient, whereas with bars, depending on their shape and design, resilient or rigid support is provided. The use of retention mechanism – resilient versus rigid – has been the subject of many discussions that rarely rely on reliable data or on a scientific background. The approach with Bonefit ITI implants is empirical as well. For support of removable prostheses that are connected to natural teeth or roots, rigid retention mechanisms are usually preferred. For anchorage of overdentures to implants, resilient retention mechanisms are widely recommended, assuming that implants will be protected from overload. Early results on force measurements with Bonefit ITI implants supporting overdentures have been published and further investigations are being undertaken.

Indications for placement of two single attachments are:

Mandible with favourable shape of the ridge, providing for denture support.

Distance between two implants that does not allow favourable design of the bar.

A resilient anchorage is preferred.

In combination with a highly reduced dentition.

Easy and most economical anchorage, where new dentures need not be made after placement of implants.

For temporary use after the healing phase and prior to the insertion of technically time consuming prosthetic reconstructions.

Contraindications are:

Maxilla and highly resorbed mandibular ridges.

Single attachments appear to require frequent adjustment, so that round or U-shaped bars in combination with Bonefit ITI implants were mostly used in the last years. It is wrong to believe that spherical attachments may be used in order to compensate for unfavourable and non-parallel placement of the implants.

Bars may be connected to two or more implants. For support of maxillary overdentures, three or four implants connected with a bar should always be prescribed. The bone structure of the maxilla is less suited than the mandible for accepting load. More failures are reported for maxillary implants. Since only few patients have been treated with maxillary implants and bars and no patients ever with single attachments, our data do not contribute to this question.

Round and U-shaped bars have regularly been used in the mandible. For support of mandibular overdentures, the placement of only two implants is adequate for most patients. With highly resorbed ridges or pronounced curvature of the man-

229

dible, three or even four implants may be advantageous. Round bars connecting two implants in a straight line provide for a resilient anchorage. The retention mechanism of round bars that follow a short curvature of the ridge between two implants or that are connected to three or more implants is likely to become rather rigid. U-shaped bars (Dolder) are always rigid and connect the implants in a straight line. Short distal extension of rigid U-shaped bars may additionally contribute to stabilize the dentures and prevent horizontal shifting. Female parts are not mounted on extensions (Figs. 9.52–9.55).

Indications for bar connectors:

Maxillary overdentures.
Atrophic residual ridges in the mandible.
Mandible with three or four implants due to pronounced curvature of the ridge.
After partial resection of soft tissue and/or bone.

Requirements for bar connectors:

To follow the shape and curvature of the ridge.
Not to interfere with the denture base and to reduce space of the intraoral cavity.
Minimal separation of implants: 10 mm.
Distal extension: $\leq$ 10 mm, not exceeding the area of the first premolars.

Maintenance

The objective of regular recalls for overdenture patients is to maintain the health of the peri-implant tissues and to check the denture with regard to fit of the base, stability, and occlusion. Maintenance in terms of prevention and of early diagnosis of problems is vital.

Patients who are elderly or who suffer impaired manual skills or reduced visual acuity are likely to experience difficulties with cleaning. Flossing will be well beyond their abilities; brushes and gauze will be more effective (Fig. 9.56). These patients require regular assistance, and individual plaque control procedures matched to each patient's ability will need to be devised.

Overdentures may enhance plaque accumulation and inflammatory soft tissue reactions. However, compared with a fixed prosthesis, the ability to remove the denture facilitates the cleaning of both implants and removable prosthesis.

Zones of problems with Bonefit ITI implants are:

- Distal and lingual sites of implants, implant shoulders.
- Lingual sides of bars.
- Soft tissue hyperplasia underneath the bar hinders optimum hygiene.
- Pseudopockets on the mesial sites of implants as a consequence of hyperplasia.
- Growth of hyperplastic soft tissue onto the implant shoulder is ob-

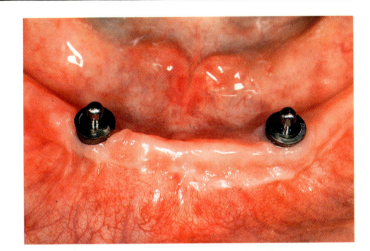

Fig. 9.52. Single spherical attachments: only to be used for mandibular dentures supported by two implants.

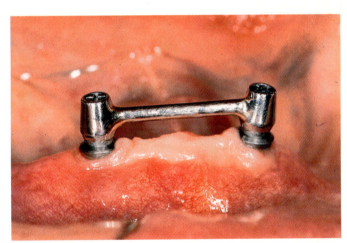

Fig. 9.53. Round bar connecting two implants in a straight line.

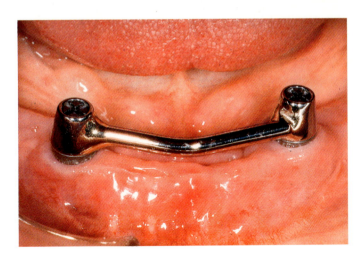

Fig. 9.54. Round bar, slightly curved, following the shape of the ridge.

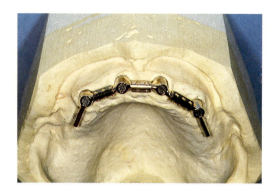

Fig. 9.55 (a). Maxillary cast: U-shaped bar with short extensions, mounted to four implants with female retainers *in situ*.

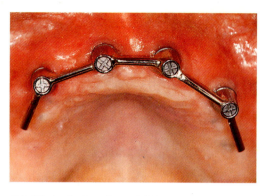

(b) Clinical situation: rigid connection of the denture is provided.

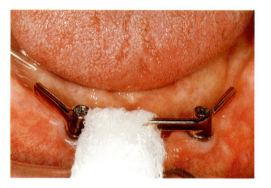

Fig. 9.56.(a) Gauze for cleaning the bar.

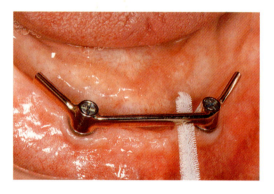

(b) Interdental brush for cleaning the approximal sites.

served with the use of Euro-abutments.

The check-up and adjustments of dentures include:
- Fit of the base, need for relining.
- Sore spots caused by the denture.
- Occlusion, need for remounting and occlusal adjustment.
- Female parts of attachments: loose, broken or lost or need to be activated.
- Wear of the gold copings by the denture base.

It is not yet known how and to what extent transfer of load to the implants might evoke resorption of bone or disintegration of osseointegrated implants. Experimental research suggests that superstructures with inadequate fit, that may even be difficult to recognize visually, may induce potentially damaging stress on implants. Precise passive fit of denture bases, bars and attachments are a prerequisite for long lasting health of the bone surrounding the implants.

10 Overdenture maintenance

Overdentures supported by roots and implants share a demanding maintenance requirement. Broadly speaking, complications, when they occur, can be divided into those affecting the supporting structures or those affecting the removable prosthesis, although the two are interrelated. For practical purposes, it is more convenient to consider root and implant supported restorations separately.

Root supported overdentures

Long-term surveys of overdentures are notable for their scarcity. Individual practitioners tend to favour particular techniques, while it is never easy to be absolutely objective about the results of one's own handiwork.

Reitz, Weiner and Levin (1977) commented that despite a high incidence of periodontal problems only one out of 50 patients had lost a support tooth. Of the 59 overdentures constructed, only one broke in use, a far lower incidence of fracture than one would normally expect. A probable cause might have been the construction technique, employing dome shaped copings or simple prepared root surfaces. The preparations occupied the minimum of space and weakened the denture less than any other overdenture technique. Sixteen percent of patients had caries and the application of topical fluoride containing solutions were considered beneficial in this respect. Periodontal complications ranged from a change in tissue tone to loss of attached gingivae and pocket formation. About 30% of the patients had abutment teeth graded as failing but, even so, these teeth could be regarded as potential abutments for a few years to come.

Over 5 years these trends appeared to have continued (Reitz, Weiner and Levin, 1980). Another 12 teeth had been extracted by this time although these teeth had demonstrated poor gingival scores at the first review. Periodontal disease was the chief cause of tooth loss. Caries of abutments did not pose a major problem. Papers by Fenton and Hahn (1978), and by Toolson and Smith (1978), highlighted the problem of caries on abutment teeth and stressed the importance of sodium fluoride gel applied at regular intervals to decrease the activity of cariogenic micro-organisms. Caries could develop in a short period of time if suitable precautions were not taken. Davis et al. (1981) stressed the periodontal factors in their 2 year longitudinal survey. They pointed out the marked difference between maxillary and mandibular teeth. While no significant decrease in attached gingivae was found in the upper teeth, a marked decrease was noted in the lower teeth. The change in width of attached gingivae was associated with an observed increase in pocket depth for mandibular teeth, whereas no significant increase in pocket depth could be found when maxillary teeth were examined. Thirty-five per cent of patients who had no gingival bleeding on probing when the dentures were first inserted showed some bleeding after the 3-year period, but there was no significant increase in tooth mobility; if anything, tooth mobility appeared to decrease. In contrast the survey of Morrow (1969) and associates showed a significant increase in pocket depth at the 2-year recall. Mandibular teeth were felt to be at greater risk than maxillary teeth. Mandibular teeth demonstrated a decrease in the width of the attached gingivae and 35% of patients who had no gingival bleeding on probing when the denture was inserted showed some bleeding after the 2-year period.

Toolson et al. (1982) found little change in attached gingivae, pocket depth or tooth mobility over a 2-year period. These investigators paid particular attention to the oral hygiene practices of their patients. Nevertheless, they did note that plaque and gingival indices were often raised but bearing in mind previous lack of motivation on the part of the patients concerned this is hardly surprising. All patients were able to wear their dentures and no teeth had been lost due to periodontal disease. These investigators commented that the effect of fluoride application on plaque prevention is uncertain, as any improvement was likely to be the result of home care rather than chemistry. They emphasised the importance of adequate follow-up care and a need for constant reinforcement of home care instruction, as few patients readily change their oral hygiene practices once the overdenture is inserted. Toolson and Smith (1983) continued their study of this same group of overdenture patients to produce a 5-year longitudinal survey although the number of patients who were able to attend had dwindled. By this time, the authors were convinced of the effectiveness of a neutral fluoride gel to control caries. The neutral pH helped to prevent tissue irritation, as it was used on a daily basis.

Pocket depth and the mobility of the retained abutments did not change significantly, although there was a loss of attached gingivae between the 2 and 5 year recall. All the patients were happy with their overdentures, while the retention and support was also maintained. This study emphasised the importance of a thorough periodontal examination of potential overdenture abutments and the motivation of patients who properly maintained their retained teeth and understood the importance of periodic examinations by the dentist.

Derkson and MacEntee (1982) showed that a 0.4% stannous fluoride gel had beneficial effects on the gingival health of overdenture abutments. It is, of course, possible that any therapeutic effect of the gel might have been potentiated by the protective environment of the overdenture base in which it has been placed.

Renner et al. (1982, 1984) were another group who focused their attention on the periodontal structures of their overdentures. These workers investigated a group of patients and made reports, 9 months, 2 years and 4 years, after the restorations were inserted. As with other workers in the field, they stressed the importance of communication skills to increase patient awareness of the problems associated with plaque control. At no time during the study were the abutments completely free of dental plaque, despite the efforts of a periodontist and dental hygienist, and a 6-monthly recall programme. As with other workers, they found statistically significant differences comparing changes in zones of attached gingivae and pocket depths around the teeth of the maxillary and mandibular arches. Although there was slight bleeding on probing of the gingival tissues, there was no overall increase of root mobility. Indeed, 25% of the roots decreased in mobility.

It is hardly surprising that workers in varying locations produce results that differ slightly. One feature they have in common is an appreciation of the sensitivity of the surrounding structures.

The encouraging results of recent investigations demonstrate the importance of proper patient selection and education, together with skilled prosthodontic therapy and maintenance. The way ahead now seems clear to provide a useful form of therapy that will benefit an ever growing section of the community.

Implant supported overdentures

Most surveys show that post-insertion maintenance for overdentures was more extensive than for fixed prostheses supported by implants. A major contributing factor, a higher implant failure rate, may be due to the fact that overdentures are often employed where insufficient volume or inadequate density of bone exists for fixed prostheses. Unpredictable loading, significant leaverages, to say nothing of the maintenance requirements of the removable section, all play a part. In a survey of 92 consecutively inserted maxillary overdentures, Jemt and others (1992) found a surprisingly high incidence of complications. They were, however, treating a group of patients with severely resorbed maxillae, in which 16% of the implants became loose and were removed. Most of the failed implants were the short 7 mm units and other workers have reported up to a 100% failure rate when short implants are employed to support maxillary overdentures. In the Jemt survey, 7 out of the 92 patients suffered complete failure of the overdenture treatment, but it must be appreciated that this was a particularly difficult group to treat.

In 1989 Kirsch reported on 143 overdentures supported by 365 IMZ implants placed in the mandible. There was a 2% failure rate of individual implants, but he claimed excellent results with bar and clip attachments provided that they were mounted parallel to the hinge axis. Over a 10-year period between 25% and 30% required rebasing, generally in the first year after insertion. Sore spots were normally found lingually, inferring a rotation around the bar. Overdentures in the maxilla should not be placed on fewer than four abutments and when the mandible is atrophic, multiple implants should be used as well.

Engquist (1991) reported on 6 years experience with overdentures involving 339 implants. There was a 30% loss of implants in the upper jaw, while the success rate in the lower jaw was 99%. The conclusions were that jaw bone quality is important. Using implant supported dentures to treat elderly patients with unfavourable maxillary jaw bone anatomy involves problems that are not yet fully understood. Correct stress distribution in relation to the total osseointegration area of supporting implants is essential. In upper jaws all the lost implants were inserted in poor quality bone or grafted jaws and that is why reducing the area of osseointegration surfaces with a short straight bar will cause lower stress with the implants but may impair denture stability, but it is possible that this bar can provide support to an implant in situations where implant length or stability is limited by jaw bone anatomy. A long curved bar may be necessary but its elasticity will then increase.

Palmquist and others (1994) are another group who stressed the pitfalls of maxillary implant supported overdentures. Provided that short implants were avoided, planned maxillary overdentures appeared to have a good prognosis. However, when these prostheses were made as an emergency procedure following loss of an implant under a fixed prosthesis, the prognosis was poor. Overdentures without palatal coverage added to the risk factors.

In the Toronto study (Zarb and others 1991), 33 patients with 35 edentulous arches participated. The Branemark system was employed. Twenty-nine of the overdentures were retained by a bar and clip assembly, two with magnets, and an overdenture and two arches were held in place with a custom designed cast framework to fit to the abutment and the acrylic resin impression surface of the denture modified to conform to the resulting contour. In the remaining two arches, a mandible and a maxilla, the overdenture was relined to accommodate the unattached abutments. One maxillary overdenture was converted to a complete denture following loss of both implants. Like all clinicians, these workers were faced with the problems of many patients with maladaptive prosthetic experience featuring bone quality and contours that would normally contraindicate implant placement. Virtually all the non-integrated implants were placed in such severely resorbed jaws, particularly maxillary ones. They also appreciated that the combination of implant and mucosal supported dentures dictated more challenging prosthodontic procedures than those encountered when making a fixed prosthesis. Later on (1994), the clinical performance of 25 mandibular implant supported overdentures was compared with 25 mandibular implant supported fixed prostheses over a 5-year period. These mandibular overdentures presented with fewer complications and maintenance requirements, doubtless due to the high standard of prosthodontics that was achieved. Like Kirsch (1991), they found that some patients required relining of their mandibular distal extension areas, suggesting that a newly acquired or renewed facility for generating forces with a stable prosthesis may elicit resorption. In fact, an opposing complete denture, when present, often required relining. Patient compliance was 100% and acceptance, together with functional and speech results, was rated as excellent. Nevertheless, a certain amount of professional maintenance is required. High on the list was adjustment of Dolder bar clips and tightening of prosthetic gold screws for the Branemark system; fractures of the Dolder bar, the gold alloy screw, and even the abutment screw were reported.

Geering (1991) reported on mandibular overdentures using the ITI system, with 56 patients receiving a total of 149 implants for mandibular overdentures. They concluded that splinting implants was unnecessary and their approach produced excellent results. They felt that the prognosis was unaffected by the choice of attachments and that for mandibular dentures two implants would suffice. McNamara and Henry (1991) found similar results to other workers using the Branemark system. In fact, their maintenance requirements were particularly high, with all the overdentures needing early relining and some being relined twice within 18 months. All subjects had problems with loosening clips and required regular maintenance. In some, the clips actually fractured and in another the entire clip loosened within the acrylic resin base. However, having experimented with magnets and stud units, these workers came to the conclusion that the bar clip was probably the most reliable.

Overdentures are both versatile and valuable methods of treatment with ever increasing applications. Long service life depends upon operator and patient understanding the maintenance requirements from the outset and the problems of maxillary implant supported prostheses must be appreciated.

Early in this text, the need to visualise the final result at the treatment planning stage was stressed. The reasons can now be understood.

Update

The recent literature concerning overdentures on implants appears to be increasing at an exponential rate, and most published work attests to the success of such restorations.

Patient satisfaction

The overwhelmingly positive response of numerous research workers worldwide should convince even the most sceptical observer. Humphris et al (1995) pointed out the psychological benefits of overdenture therapy. Those with the greatest amount of bone loss derived the maximum benefit. In a cross over study Burns et al (1995) showed that edentulous patients preferred an overdenture to a complete denture. Of the overdenture designs the O-ring proved more popular than the magnet.

Surveys

An impressive number of prospective and retrospective studies confirm the high success rate that can be achieved with a variety of implant systems (Hutton et al 1995 and Preiskel, Tsolka 1995). Of note was the higher failure rate of maxillary implants and overdentures compared with their mandibular counterparts. One multicentre study reported the ratio as 9:1. It is apparent that subjects with the highest risk of failure are those requiring maxillary restorations with limited bone of poor density. Short implants (7mm) to support maxillary overdentures appear to have an unacceptable failure rate. Inflammation of the peri-implant tissues was more common with maxillary overdentures. Most, but not all, workers found the maintenance requirements of overdentures greater than that of fixed prostheses.

Jemt and Lekholm (1995) suggested that treatment outcomes with edentulous maxillae might be predicted by careful presurgical evaluation of jaw shape. Patients provided with autogenous bone grafts compared favourably with the group presenting severely resorbed jaws.

Quirynen et al (1991) noted that loaded lower jaw implants connected by a straight bar had a radiographic bone loss of 0.8mm during the first post surgical year followed by a mean annual bone loss of less than 0.1mm. However, loaded but unconnected implants in the upper jaw demonstrated 2.0mm loss during the first six months which might raise questions about the wisdom of using unconnected implants in the maxilla. As for the mandible Naert et al (1994) found no clinical difference between overdentures on splinted and unsplinted implants but stressed this was a short term observation requiring longer term data.

Donatsky (1993) published a survey of patients suffering from mandibular alveolar ridge atrophy who had been treated with overdentures supported by ball attachments. The success rates of the individual implants (97%) and of the dentures (100%) were impressive.

Occlusal forces and masticatory efficiency

A number of studies confirm that patients with implant supported overdentures apply greater loads and chew more efficiently than their edentulous counterparts. The mechanism of this improvement is not so clear cut. Geertman et al (1994) suggested that increased stability and support was the important factor. While the mean peak masticatory force varies considerably from subject to subject the forces appear consistent for each subject (Hobkirk et al 1992).

When comparing overdentures supported by roots and those supported by implants Mericske-Stern et al (1993 a.) found greater powers of discrimination among the group with roots, whereas there was a tendency for patients with implant supported overdentures to chew slightly harder. In another study (1993 b.) no differences between implant angulation and function could be found. Masticatory patterns (Mericske-Stern et al 1992) demonstrated a dominating vertical component. Jemt et al (1993) noted a decrease in occlusal force when the bar of an overdenture was removed although this removal would have influenced the support, stability and retention. However, both Jemt (1995) and Jacobs et al (1995) suggested that patients with fixed prostheses might apply higher loading to the structure than those with overdentures. Load is defined as an externally applied force or moment which is responsible for an internal stress condition in the material. Stresses in the surrounding tissues are a consequence of loading implants. Stress distribution in the bone surrounding implants can only be estimated by models. Of the various studies undertaken the highest stresses in bone were normally located around the neck of the implant. With mandibular prostheses the direction of the force had more influence on stress distribution than the connection of implant abutments (Chao et al 1995). Nevertheless it is clear that patients with implant supported and retained overdentures derive considerable benefit and apply more load than those who are edentulous. The structures to which these loads are applied must be able to withstand them; implant therapy is no substitute for poor prosthodontics. While the mean peak masticatory force varies considerably from subject to subject the forces appear consistent for each subject (Hobkirk et al 1992). The force as in chewing should simulate the force during mastication but there is doubt if the measurements are reliable in this respect.

Innovative techniques

Using spark erosion technology allows for the production of closely adapted removable sections that can combine the versatility of overdentures with the effectiveness of fixed prostheses (Salonen et al 1994). However, a corresponding increase in the amount of implant support is required that will limit their application. Connecting implants with bars may well have mechanical advantages but carries with it the potential inaccuracies of castings and soldering techniques remote from the mouth on casts that may not be entirely accurate reproductions. Hruska and Borelli (1993) have described a method of intraoral welding while Mazurat and Love (1993) employed a resin based approach to unite the components. It can now be seen that overdentures on implants have proved their place

in the prosthodontic armamentarium.

The versatility and effectiveness of these devices should not be allowed to overshadow the difficulties of design, construction, and maintenance. The maxillary overdenture can play such an important role in the restoration of the facial skeleton yet provides the greatest difficulties in construction and maintenance. Developments are inevitable, bounded only by the imagination and skill of the prosthodontists.
Master the simple — the rest will follow!

References

Burns D.R., Unger J.W., Elswick R.K.Jr., Beck D.A. Prospective clinical evaluation of mandibular implant overdentures: Part I Retention, stability, and tissue response. J. Prosthet. Dent. 73(4): 354-63 1995

Chao Y.L., Meijer H.J.M., van Oort R.P., Veersteegh P.A.M. The incomprehensible success of the implant stabilised overdenture in the edentulous mandible: A literature review on transfer of chewing forces to bone implants. (Lower implant stabilised Overdentures only) European J. Prosthod. and Rest. Dent. 3: 6: 225-260 1995

Donatsky O. Osseointegrated dental implants with ball attachments supporting overdentures in patients with mandibular alveolar ridge atrophy. Int. J. Oral Maxillofac. Impl. 8(2): 162-6 1993

Geertman M.E., Slagter A.P., van Waas M.A., Kalk W. Comminution of food with mandibular implant-retained overdentures. J. Dent. Res. 73(12): 1858-64 1994

Hopkirk J.A., Psarros K.J. The influence of occlusal surface material on peak masticatory force using osseointegrated implant-supported prostheses. Int. J. Oral. Maxillofac. Impl. 7: 345-352 1992

Hruska A.R., Borelli P. Intro-oral welding of implants for an immediate load with overdentures. J. Oral Implant. 19(1): 34-8 1993

Hutton J.E., Heath M.R., Chai J.Y., Harnett J., Jemt T., Johns R.B., McKenna S., McNamara D.C., van Steenberghe D., Taylor R., et al. Factors related to success and failure rates at 3-year follow-up in a multicenter study of overdentures supported by Branemark implants. Int. J. Oral Maxillofac. Impl. 10(1): 33-42 1995

Humphris G.M., Healey T., Howell R.A., Cawood J. The psychological impact of implant-retained mandibular prostheses: a cross-sectional study. Int. J. Oral Maxillofac. Impl. 10(4): 437-44 1995

Jacobs R., van Steenberghe D., Naert I. Masseter muscle fatigue before and after rehabilitation with implant-supported prostheses. J. Prosthet. Dent. 73(3): 284-9 1995

Jemt T., Book K., Karlsson S. Occlusal force and mandibular movements in patients with removable overdentures and fixed prostheses supported by implants in the maxilla. J. Oral Maxillofac. Impl. 8(3): 301-8 1993

Jemt T., Lekholm U. Implant treatment in edentulous maxillae: a 5-year follow-up report on patients with different degrees of jaw resorption. Int. J. Oral Maxillofac. Impl. 10(3): 303-11 1995

Mazurat R.D., Love W.B. Direct assembly of implant suprastructures. J. Prosthet. Dent. 70(2): 172-5 1993

Mericske-Stern R., Geering A.H., Burgin W.B., Graf H. Three-dimensional force measurements on mandibular implants supporting overdentures. Int. J. Oral Maxillofac. Impl. 7(2): 195-94 1992

Mericske-Stern R. Forces on implants supporting overdentures: a preliminary study of morphologic and cephalometric considerations. Int. J. Oral Maxillofac. Impl. 8(3): 254-63 1993 a

Mericske-Stern R., Hofmann J., Wedig A., Geering A.H. In vivo measurements of maximal occlusal force and minimal pressure threshold on overdentures supported by implants or natural roots: a comparative study, Part 1. Int. J. Oral Maxillofac. Impl. 8(6): 641-9 1993 b

Naert I., Quirynen M., Hooghe M., van Steenberghe D. A comparative prospective study of splinted and unsplinted Branemark implants in mandibular overdenture therapy: a preliminary report. J. Prosthet. Dent. 71(5): 486-92 1994

Preiskel H.W., Tsolka P. Treatment outcomes in implant therapy: the influence of surgical and prosthodontic experience. Int. J. Prosthet. 8: 3: 273-279 1995

Salonen M.A., Oikarinen K.S., Raustia A.M., Knuuttila M., Virtanen K.K. Clinical and radiologic assessment of possibilities for endosseous implants and osseointegrated prostheses in 55 year-old edentulous subjects. Acta. Odont. Scand. 52(1): 25-32 1994

Quirynen M., Naert I., van Steenberghe D., Teerlinck J., Dekeyser C., Theuniers G. Periodontal aspects of osseointegrated fixtures supporting an overdenture. A 4-year retrospective study. J. Clin. Periodont. 18(10): 719-28 1991

Zarb G.A., Schmitt A. Osseointegration and the edentulous predicament. The 10 year old Toronto study. Brit. Dent. J. 170(12): 439-44 1991

242

Bibliography

Textbooks

Bates J.F., Neill D.J., Preiskel H.W. Restoration of the Partially Dentate Mouth: Proceedings of the International Prosthodontic Symposium. Quintessence, Chicago 1984

Basker R.M., Harrison A., Ralph J.P., Watson C.J. Overdentures in general dental practice. 3rd Ed. B.D.J. 1994

Brewer A.A., Morrow R.M. Overdentures. 2nd Ed. C.V. Mosby Co., St Louis 1980

Essig C.J. The American Textbook of Prosthetic Dentistry. Lea and Febiger, Philadelphia p. 439 1896

Neill D.J., Nairn R.I. Complete Denture Prosthetics. 3rd Ed. Wright, London 1990

Preiskel H.W. Precision Attachments in Prosthodontics: Overdentures and telescopic prostheses. Vol. 2. Quintessence, Chicago 1985

Schepers E., Naert I., Theuniers G. (Co-Editors). Overdentures on Oral Implants: Proceedings of the symposium on implant supported overdentures: November 1989, Brussels. Leuven University Press 1991

Root Supported Overdentures

Atkinson W.H. Plates over Fangs. Dent. Reg. 1861 15: 213-216

Atwood D.A., Coy W.A. Clinical cephalometric and densitometric study of reduction of residual ridges. J. Prosthet. Dent. 1971 26: 3: 280-299

Bennett A.G. The vertical half-cap or bridgework anchorage. Dent. Cosmos 1904: 46: 367

Bolender C.L., Smith D.E., Toolson L.B. Overdentures: their effectiveness and clinical considerations in treating the partially dentate mouth. In: Restoration of the Partially Dentate Mouth: Proceedings of the International Prosthodontic Symposium. Quintessenz, Berlin 1984

Budtz-Jorgensen E. Effect of controlled oral hygiene in overdenture wearers: A 3-year study. Int. J. Prosthodont. 1991: 4: 226-231

Budtz-Jorgensen E., Thylstrup A. The effect of controlled oral hygiene in overdenture wearers. Acta Odontol. Scand. 1988: 46: 219-225

Carr C.M. Anchored adjustable dentures. Dent. Cosmos 1898 40: 219

Crum R.J., Rooney G.E. Alveolar bone loss in overdentures: A 5-year study. J. Prosthet. Dent. 1978 40: 6: 610-613

Davis R.K., Renner R.D., Antos E.W., Schlissel E.R., Baer P.N. Two year longitudinal study of periodontal health status of overdenture patients. J. Prosthet. Dent. 1981 45: 4: 358-363

Derkson G.D., MacEntee, M.M. Effect of 0.4% stannous fluoride gel on the gingival health of overdenture abutments. J. Prosthet. Dent. 1982 48: 1: 23-26

Ettinger R. Overdentures: A Longitudinal Perspective. D. Sc. Thesis University of Sydney 1990

Ettinger R.L., Taylor T.D., Scandrett F.R. Treatment needs of overdenture patients in a longitudinal study: Five-year results. J. Prosthet. Dent. 1984 52: 4: 532-536

Ettinger R.L. Tooth loss in an overdenture population. J. Prosthet. Dent. 1988 60: 4: 459-462

Ettinger R.L., Manderson D., Wefel J.S., Jensen M.E. An in-vitro evaluation of the prevention of caries on overdenture abutments. J. Dent. Res. 1988 67: 1338-1341

Ettinger R.L., Jakobsen J. Caries: a problem in an overdenture population. Community Dent. Oral Epidemiol. 1990: 18: 42-45

Fenton A.H., Hahn N. Tissue response to overdenture therapy. J. Prosthet. Dent. 1978 40: 5: 492-498

Gilmore S.F. A method of retention. Council of Allied Dental Societies 1913 8: 118

Gillings B.R.D. Magnetic Denture Retention Systems: In: Preiskel H.W. Precision Attachments in Prosthodontics: Overdentures and telescopic prostheses. Vol. 2. Quintessence, Chicago 1985

Goslee H.J. Removable bridgework. Dent. Items Interest 1912 34: 731

Hunter W. Oral sepsis in relation to disease. Brit. J. Dent. Sc. 1906 4711: 805

Kawamura Y. Watanabe M. Studies in oral sensory thresholds. Med. J. Osaka Univ. 1960 10: 291

Ledger E. On preparing the mouth for the reception of a full set of artificial teeth. Br. J. Dent. Sc. 1856. 1: 90

Lord J.L., Teel S. The overdenture. Dent. Clin. N. Amer. 1969 13: 871-881

Lord J.L., Teel S. The overdenture: patient selection, use of copings and follow-up evaluation. J. Prosthet. Dent. 1974 32: 1: 41-51

Miller P.A. Complete dentures supported by natural teeth. J. Prosthet. Dent. 1958 8: 6: 924-928

Morrow R.M., Feldman E.E., Rudd K.D., Howard H.J. Tooth supported complete dentures. An approach to preventive prosthodontics. J. Prosthet. Dent. 1969 21: 5: 513-522

Reitz P.V., Weiner M.G., Levin B. An overdenture survey. Preliminary report. J. Prosthet. Dent. 1977 37: 246

Reitz, P., Weiner M.N., Levin B. An overdenture survey: second report. J. Prosthet. Dent. 1980 43: 4: 457-462

Renner R.P., Gomes B.C., Shakun M.L., Baer P.N. Camp P. Four-year longitudinal study of the periodontal health status of overdenture patients. J. Prosthet. Dent. 51: 5: 593 1984

Tallgren A. The effect of denture wearing on facial morphology: A 7-year longitudinal study. Acta. Odont. Scand. 1967 25: 563-592

Tallgren A. Positional changes of complete dentures: A 7-year longitudinal study. Acta. Odont. Scand. 1969 27: 539

Tallgren A., Walker G.F., Lang B.R., Holder S., Ash M.M. Cephalometric analysis of ridge resorption and changes in jaw and occlusal relationships in denture wearers. J. Dent. Res. 1978 57: 907

Thayer H.H., Caputo A.A. Effects of overdentures on remaining oral structures. J. Prosthet. Dent. 1977 37: 4: 374-381

Thayer H.H., Caputo A.A. Occlusal force transmission by overdentures. In: Brewer A.A., Morrow R.M. Overdentures. 2nd ed. C.V. Mosby, St Louis 1980

Toolson L.B., Smith D.E. A two year longitudinal study of overdenture patients. Part I: Incidence and control of caries on overdenture abutments. J. Prosthet. Dent. 1978 40: 486

Toolson L.B., Smith D.E., Phillips C. A two-year longitudinal study of overdenture patients. Part II: Assessment of the periodontal health of overdenture abutments. J. Prosthet. Dent. 1982 47: 1: 4-11

Toolson, L.B., Smith D.E. A five-year longitudinal study of patients treated with overdentures. J. Prosthet. Dent. 1983 49: 6: 749

Overdentures on Implants

Engquist B., Bergendal T., Kallus T., Linden U. A retrospective multicenter evaluation of osseointegrated implants supporting overdentures. Int. J. Oral Maxillofac. Implants 1988: 3: 129-134

Engquist B. Six years experience of splinted and non-splinted implants supporting overdentures in upper and lower jaws. In: Overdentures on Oral Implants: Proceedings of symposium on implant supported overdentures. November 1989, Brussels. Leuven University Press 1991

Geering A.H. Mandibular overdentures on ITI implants. In: Overdentures on Oral Implants: Proceedings of the symposium on implant supported overdentures: November 1989, Brussels. Leuven University Press 1991

Hemmings K.W., Schmitt A., Zarb G.A. Complications and maintenance requirements for fixed prostheses in the edentulous mandible: A 5-year report. Int. J. Oral Maxillofac. Implants 1994 9: 2: 191

Jempt T., Book K., Linden B., Urde G. Failures and complications in 92 consecutively inserted overdentures supported by Branemark implants in severely resorbed edentulous maxillae: A study from prosthetic treatment to first annual check-up. Int. J. Oral Maxillofac. Implants 1992 7: 162-167

Jempt T., Stalblad P.A. The effect of chewing movements on changing mandibular complete dentures to osseointegrated overdentures. J. Prosthet. Dent. 1986 55: 3: 357-361

Johns R.B. Overdenture treatment with the Branemark implant. In Albrektsson T., Zarb G.A. (eds). The Branemark Osseointegrated Implant pp 215-220. Quintessence, Chicago 1989

Johns R.B., Jempt T., Heath M.R., Hutton J.E., McNamara D.C., Van Steenberghe D., Taylor R., Watson R.M., Herrmann I. A multicentre study of overdentures supported by Branemark implants. Int. J. Oral Maxillofac Implants 1992: 7: 513-522

Kirsch A., Overdentures on IMZ implants: Modalities and long-term results. In: Overdentures on Oral Implants. Proceedings of the symposium on implant supported overdentures. November 1989, Brussels. Leuven University Press 1991

Lindquist L.W., Carlsson G.E. Changes in masticatory function in complete denture wearers after insertion of bridges on osseointegrated implants in the lower jaw. Adv. Biomaterials 1982 4: 151-155

McNamara D. Osseointegrated overdentures with bar/clip retention. In: Overdentures on Oral Implants. Proceedings of the symposium on implant supported overdentures. November 1989, Brussels. Leuven University Press 1991

Palmquist S. Sondell K. Implant supported maxillary overdentures: Outcome in planned and emergency cases. Int. J. of Oral Maxillofac. Implants 1994 9: 2: 184

Stalblad P.A., Jansson T., Jempt T., Zarb G. Osseointegration in overdenture therapy. Swed. Dent. J. 1985 Suppl. 28: 169-170

Zarb G. The Toronto overdenture study: Interim conclusions. In: Overdentures on Oral Implants: Proceedings of the symposium on implant supported overdentures. November 1989, Brussels. Leuven University Press 1991

Index